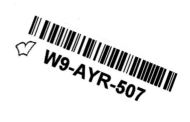

CANCER
is a *word*
not a *sentence*

CANCER
is a *word*
not a *sentence*

a practical guide

to help you through

the first few weeks

Dr. Robert Buckman

With Major Contributions by Dr. Pamela Catton
and the Medical Staff of the Princess Margaret Hospital

FIREFLY BOOKS

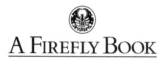

A FIREFLY BOOK

Published by Firefly Books Ltd. 2006

First printing

Publisher Cataloging-in-Publication Data (U.S.)

Buckman, Robert.
  Cancer is a word, not a sentence : a practical guide to help you through the first few weeks / Robert Buckman.
[280]p. : cm.
Includes index.
Summary: A practical guide for people diagnosed with cancer, including tests, the stages of the disease, treatment options, follow-up and daily life.
ISBN-13: 978-1-55407-234-7 (pbk.)
ISBN-10: 1-55407-234-4 (pbk.)
1. Cancer – popular works. I. Title.
616.99/ 4 dc22   RC263.B835 2006

Published in the United States by
Firefly Books (U.S.) Inc.
P.O. Box 1338, Ellicott Station
Buffalo, New York 14205

Published in Canada by
Key Porter Books Ltd.
6 Adelaide St. East, 10th Floor
Toronto, Ontario M5C 1H6

Cover and text design: Marijke Friesen
Electronic formating: Jean Lightfoot Peters

Printed in Canada

This book is dedicated with deep, genuine respect and admiration to a man who combines careful research, vision and foresight with extraordinary compassion and humanity:

DR. JUDAH FOLKMAN

AUTHOR'S NOTE

I am indebted to the Macmillan Cancer Relief charity of Great Britain, where I first heard "Cancer is a word, not a sentence" used in 2002. As I thought about it afterwards, it occurred to me that the phrase identifies precisely the entire problem caused by the overtones and the shades of meaning associated with the word cancer. —RB

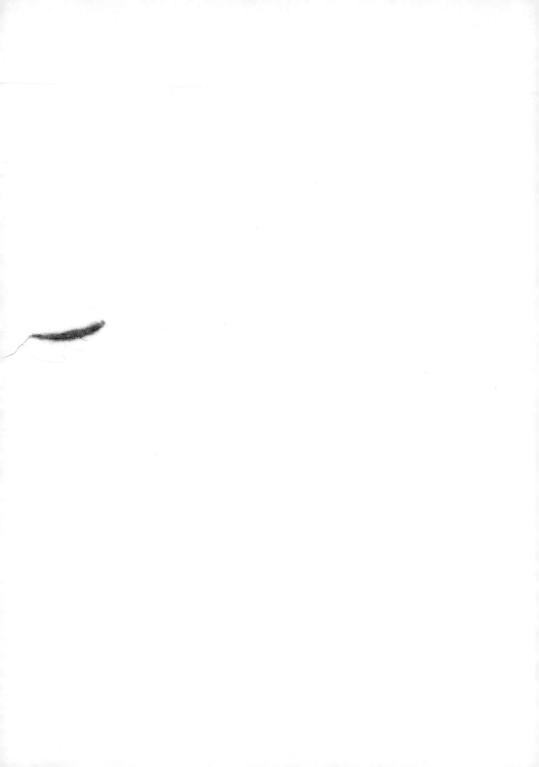

TABLE OF CONTENTS

A Word,
Not a Sentence

Read This First–It Will Help You Get Your Balance Back

If you're reading this book, you're probably reeling.

Almost everybody is knocked off balance and is reeling when the diagnosis is a cancer. It's the normal reaction: it's what everybody experiences, and it's why I've written this particular book, with the collaboration of my friend and colleague Dr. Pam Catton and many other members of the medical staff of the Princess Margaret Hospital, in this particular way.

This book is going to do one specific thing for you: it's going to help you get your balance back. It will do that by offering a steady hand that guides you and gives you a sense of direction.

The problem starts with the word *cancer*. There are so many overtones and associations attached, it is probably the most dreaded word in the English language. It brings with it, universally, queasy feelings of fear and doom. Many people describe the sensation as chilling, or as a sense of helplessness, or even as a foggy feeling of mental paralysis. They experience a sense of unreality, and feel "this can't be happening to me."

That's why I wrote this book: to help you get over that initial shock and to understand, make sense of, and then cope with the facts of your own situation. I wrote this book, in fact, to help you get your balance back.

A Simple Fact of Unparalleled Importance

Let's start that balance-restoring process with a simple fact—and it's a fact that I think everybody *should* know, but which most don't.

It might be the most ignored and under-publicized medical statistic in the known world!

It is this: *of all the people diagnosed with one of the cancers this year, just over half will survive it and will not be troubled by it for the rest of their life.*

I think that's worth repeating. If you have one of the cancers, over-all—that is, taking all the cases diagnosed this year in the whole country—the chance of surviving it (and, in most uses of the word, being considered cured) is approximately 50 percent.

That's not as high a percentage as it should be—90 or even 100 percent would be better. But that figure, which has been increasing steadily over the last four or five decades, is vastly better than what most people think it is, or fear it might be.

Even though we live in an age in which we are awash with information, that one fact seems to have remained submerged. Many people still think that a diagnosis of a cancer *is* a sentence.

One of my patients put it succinctly: "We all have this feeling that if we're diagnosed with a cancer on Monday we'll be dead by Wednesday. Thursday at the latest. If we're lucky."

That is what most people have in the backs of their minds, and that is why it is so difficult to cope with any cancer diagnosis. Even when you are told that the prognosis is good—let's say for a small cancer of the breast that has not spread to the lymph nodes—you will most likely still have a deep-seated doubt, a tendency not to believe that news.

That's why this book is necessary, and why I've given it such a specific title. The whole problem starts with the fact that we are discussing a word, a single word that (as you'll see) lumps together over two hundred different diseases. Yet that word should not be the end of a conversation, it should be a beginning—it should be the start of a fact-finding mission. As you will learn in the rest of this book, what really matters to you is not simply the diagnosis itself, but many other aspects of your situation that are much more important and relevant to you and your future.

Questions such as these:

What specific disease—which of the two hundred different cancers—is it?
What does it actually mean for your future?
How does this particular cancer behave?
What are the treatment options?

By beginning to answer those questions you will start to get a picture of what is going on in your case, and that's what you need in order to begin coping with your situation.

The word *cancer* is the start to finding out, as precisely as possible, and with more and more accuracy over time, what is going on. As the title of this book tells you from the get-go, *cancer* is just a word. It's not a sentence.

The Map with the "You Are Here" Sticker

You need to get your sense of direction back, too.

A general sense of direction—knowing the way the land lies and the way things are going—helps you get back some feeling of control.

Most people—not everyone, but most—find that one of the really difficult aspects of a new cancer diagnosis is the feeling that they've lost control. You haven't got a clear overall picture of the situation: you feel bewildered and "de-skilled." To make matters worse, many of the new people that you meet in your medical team may not have the time to explain the big picture to you. Sometimes they do, and when that happens you're lucky. But there is a lot to do and organize at the time of diagnosis, staging, and the start of treatment. And clinics are generally extremely busy places. In most cases the time to explain the overview simply isn't there. That's another reason why there seems to be a real need for this guidebook.

In a way, what I am doing here is creating a cancer-treatment map, like the ones you see in the entrances to shopping malls with a bright yellow "You Are Here" sticker to give you a sense of direction. I hope that this book will provide you with your own bright yellow sticker and will, in a perplexing and complicated territory, give you some idea of where you are and where the various paths and options lead.

So this book is intended to fill a gap. Most of the current books about cancer give you the relevant facts and usually discuss treatment options. Obviously you're going to need that kind of information as well. (And you'll find it in the companion volume to this one, *What You Really Need to Know About Cancer.*) But as you first come to grips with a diagnosis of one of the cancers, you need something else. You need a practical guide that matches your day-to-day experience.

This book is, I hope, precisely that. It is the first step-by-step "what-do-I-do-now," practical guide specifically written to help you through those first few bewildering weeks and the various steps of diagnosis and treatment, and to provide simple, practical, everyday help in coping.

So what you'll find here is not a comprehensive compilation of cancer facts, biology, and treatment. (That's all in *What You Really Need to Know About Cancer.*) Instead, you'll find a clear and straightforward guide for use in your real world. It will show you what the diagnosis actually means, what the tests are all about, what the future depends on, how to judge the benefits of various treatment options, and how to cope with the side effects of treatment and all the various uncertainties and ups and downs of follow-up. In simple and straightforward language this book explains what's happening and how to cope with it.

You need something that shows you how this new and unfamiliar terrain is laid out, and gives you some sense of direction as you navigate your way through it.

When you're lost in a forest, you don't need a catalog of the trees. You need a map of the forest.

The Bottom Line at the Top of the Book

So right at the start, let me give you a few simple guidelines. I'll explain more about them as we go along, but we all like a hint of the bottom line upfront, so here are the most important dos and don'ts:

SOME IMPORTANT DOS, SOME IMPORTANT DON'TS

Do try to get a reasonable, general overview of your type of cancer.	**Don't** respond simply to the word "cancer" as a universal and total signal of doom and gloom.
Do get a small amount of trustworthy current information: perhaps visit a few reputable cancer Web sites (see Appendix B on page 269) or/and have a look at the companion volume to this one, *What You Really Need to Know About Cancer.*	**Don't** go to the Internet and collect hundreds of different views, opinions, home remedies, and fringe medications. By and large if there really is something major going on, almost all the professionals know about it.
Do accept, which means admit and acknowledge to yourself, any uncertainty about the diagnosis and/or treatment at this stage. Uncertainty is always unpleasant—and it's easier to cope with if you acknowledge that fact.	**Don't** think that things won't change after you hear the first view of the diagnosis or treatment. Plans may well change as time goes on, so try to stay as flexible as possible.
Do ask your medical team a few specific questions once you understand the general overview of your situation	**Don't**—or try not to—ask the same questions too often. Two or three times are usually enough. Asking over and over again usually means that it's difficult for you to accept the answers.
Do get a second opinion if you really think you need it.	**Don't** get a third opinion (or more!) if the second opinion is the same as the first.
Do think about why you want to go to a complementary medicine remedy or clinic and what you expect.	**Don't** make a major early investment (in time, money, or hope) in complementary medicine or a clinic without thinking about it for a time and discussing it.
Do take a few minutes to look at the ways you can talk to your medical team and your friends.	**Don't** shout at your friends and family, or blame them. (Or try not to, anyway.) It's usually better to explain your feelings, rather than exhibit them, although we all have some moments when we can only vent.

Do talk to your friends and family.	**Don't** feel that you have to hold all your concerns and worries in until you know all the answers.
Do tell the people you like that you like them. Nobody minds being told nice things!	**Don't** cut yourself off from the people that you really like. We all tend to feel a bit uneasy and vulnerable when things aren't going well or we are upset. True friends are people you can share those feelings with.
Do Breathe! With the word "cancer" most people have a feeling that the roof will fall in tomorrow. This book is all about dispelling that illusion.	**Don't Panic!** The word "cancer" causes in almost everyone a major sense of urgency and panic. In the vast majority of situations, even though it's difficult to believe, there is plenty of time to get informed and make decisions.
Do spend a little bit of time every day doing something you really enjoy and thus look forward to. It can be any-thing, even watching a favorite TV program or listening to a CD.	**Don't** sell the furniture! Which is the same thing as Don't Panic—a motto that's so important it's worth saying twice.

I Keep on Wondering..."

Many people find that they have dozens of questions running through their minds when they are given a diagnosis of cancer. The two most frequent questions which go round and round in their thoughts are:

What does this diagnosis *actually* mean in my case?
What's going to happen? (In other words, what does the future hold?)

Often, you may find that those questions can't be answered with certainty. With the best will in the world, even the most experienced clinician can't predict precisely what is going to happen to every single person with a cancer, or how every individual case is going to turn out.

But it is often possible to explain in general terms what the situation looks like, and which aspects of the tumor have the greatest bearing on what's likely to happen.

So the whole point of this book is to show you the path that you'll travel in the first few weeks, and to make sense of the various tests and of the several uncertainties that you're likely to encounter along that path. I hope that this guide will help you make sense of what's going on.

Understanding Is the Beginning of Coping

Getting your balance back is the start: and it's the beginning of a process by which you build up your own coping strategies—the personal psychological mechanisms and devices that you use (as do we all) to cope with shocks and bad news.

By the time you've read through this book you'll find that you can put your own personal diagnosis and medical plan into some form of perspective. A cancer diagnosis almost always makes you feel overwhelmed, often helpless, and almost paralyzed at first. The information, hints and tips in this guide will make it easier for you to understand what's going on and how to cope with it.

When it comes to coping with cancer, the cure for that nasty feeling of paralysis is understanding. And that's the whole idea of this book. It's the first stop on the way to getting your situation into perspective and putting your own "You Are Here" sticker on the map.

A Guide to This Guide

This book consists of this introductory chapter, six Parts, a section of Tables, and an appendix.

Part One, "What's Going to Happen to Me Next?" is the equivalent of the large-scale map of the main highways. It gives you the broad overview of how things are arranged, and how they happen.

In Part One I start by explaining the basics: what cancer actually is (or rather, what the cancer process actually is), and how the cancer process is a feature common to the two hundred or more different diseases that we call *the cancers*. I also explain that most of those different diseases have little in common with each other, apart from sharing the basic cancer process.

After that, I set out the six basic steps of planning and coping, from the moment of diagnosis onward. This part is basically the map of how cancers are diagnosed, assessed, and then treated, with explanations of why follow-up is so important and how to cope with the anxiety it often produces.

What you will find there are clear and straightforward explanations of the various (often mystifying and bewildering) tests, results, discussions, treatment plans, and so on; and also a detailed strategy for asking the right questions to get a real understanding of your situation.

Part Two, "What's Treatment Like?" explains the four main types of treatment used in treating the cancers—surgery, radiotherapy, chemotherapy and biologic agents—and explains how treatment is constantly being improved by research studies called *clinical trials*. This part concludes with some practical tips about communicating with your medical team: who the various members are, and some guidelines for discussing potentially awkward situations, such as your feelings and requests for a second opinion.

Part Three, "Isn't There an Easier Way?" deals with complementary medicine. It will help you weigh and assess the many alluring claims made for remedies that are said to be active in treating cancers while not producing side effects. I believe that it is very important to think clearly about *why* you want to try complementary remedies and what you might expect from them.

Part Four, the all-important "How Do I Get Back on Track?" is all about recovering: getting back to normal, or nearly, after and during treatment. Here you will find some general guidelines to help you restore some order and balance to your life, plus a section on how to talk with other people, including your friends and relatives. I have also included a section specifically for your family and friends, setting out some guidelines on how to talk to you.

Part Four continues with discussions of spirituality and religion, and then sexuality and dealing with sexual problems that are quite common after cancer diagnosis and treatment. It concludes with a section on hope: what it means and the many different forms it can take.

Part Five, "Do I Always Have to Have a Positive Attitude?" deals with a widely debated topic: cancer and the mind. Here you will find a discussion of the many claims and statements made about the effect of the mind on the cancer process itself, including a review of several major studies which have been done on this subject.

Part Six is called "What Can I Do to Help Myself?" and you will be glad to know that the first section of this part is called "You've Already Started." Here, I summarize the process of regaining control over what seems at first an arbitrary and uncontrollable situation, and I conclude this part with the most important statement about the value of support: *you are not alone.*

Then, the section of Tables provides detailed descriptions of various drugs, tests, and procedures.

Finally, in Appendix B on page 269 you will find a list of national organizations and their phone numbers and Web sites, plus some other Internet sources that are trustworthy and credible.

"What's Going to Happen to Me Next?"

A Step-by-Step Guide

Beginning at the Beginning: What Is Cancer Anyway?

Curiously enough, cancer is not a disease.

Everyone uses the word as if it represents one disease, in the same way we refer to diabetes, multiple sclerosis, or Alzheimer's as diseases. But cancer is not a single disease at all—it is a *process*. It is a process by which many different diseases—the cancers—are created. And that fact, as you will see, changes everything.

Cancer or The Cancers? A Big Difference

Let me start by stating that main point again: cancer is not a disease, it is a process. Furthermore, that process is shared by over two hundred very different diseases—such as cancer of the breast, cancer of the lung, cancer of the bowel and so on—which together make up a widely disparate group that we should really call *the cancers*. The central point—and this is important—is that most cancers have very little in common with each other, apart from sharing the fundamental cancer process.

Let's take a couple of examples to illustrate the very wide range of conditions that make up the cancers. (This may sound a bit simplistic, but stay with me: it's a very important point.)

If you have had one of the common types of skin cancer—basal cell cancer, or the other common type, squamous cell cancer—once the lesion has been removed, it is highly unlikely that the cancer will ever cause you any trouble again. You may later develop other skin cancers on other parts of your body, and occasionally the cancer can come back in its original place, but it is exceptionally rare for anyone to be seriously affected by one of these types of skin cancer. These particular cancers never spread to distant or important parts of your body, and so they never pose a threat to your life. It's that simple.

In fact, from the point of view of endangering your health or life, it would almost be possible, as a patient once put it so neatly, to think of these types of cancer in the same way we think of warts—which are themselves benign tumors, growths that do not invade or spread.

For that very reason these types of skin cancer—as opposed to the much rarer melanoma, which may in some circumstances recur or spread—are not included in the cancer statistics. So when we are told that approximately 150,000 new cases of all types of cancer will be diagnosed in Canada this year, and about 1.2 million in the United States, those numbers do *not* include the common skin cancers, which in themselves probably number several million cases. In many respects, then, the common skin cancers represent one end of the spectrum: they are cancers, but once they are removed the chance of their causing you serious trouble is zero.

On the other hand, if you happen to have, let's say, advanced cancer of the pancreas, the chance of it being cured is very low. Pancreatic cancer is always very serious, and it has a high probability of threatening your life.

These two examples—skin and pancreas—in many ways represent the two ends of the spectrum. They behave in totally different ways and have nothing in common with each other, apart from the cancer process itself. They are not the same disease in any way.

Now, this is not just a matter of semantics or grammar. The language that we use and the way we use it deeply affects the way we think. And *that* changes the way we feel—and how worried or afraid we may be when any topic is raised. That effect is particularly evident—and very powerful—with the cancers. The way we think and talk about this group of diseases greatly affects the impact that we usually feel when we hear a diagnosis including the word *cancer*.

This point is so important that I want to take it a little further. The general view that cancer is a single terrible disease is now so ingrained into our way of thinking that it's quite difficult for us to think differently. But it is so important for you to get rid of the old cancer-is-a-single-disease idea, that I would like to use another analogy to illustrate the point. So let's look at what would happen if you took another large group of diseases, the infectious diseases, and lumped *them* all together, as if they were one single disease.

"Cancer" as Compared to "Infection"

As we all know, the infectious diseases cover a vast spectrum of seriousness, from the totally trivial to the lethal. At the trivial end of the spectrum is the common cold. We've all had colds. We all know that a cold is caused by a virus, of the type known as a rhinovirus, infecting the lining of the nose. We sniff and snuffle for a few days, then it goes away and we forget about it.

Now think about another example of a virus infecting an organ and causing trouble: hepatitis B. Hepatitis B is an infection of the liver that is unpleasant and can sometimes be very serious. Then there are other viruses that are even more serious—for example Ebola virus or Marburg virus (both of which have very high mortality rates), HIV/AIDS, or avian flu.

We would not dream of grouping these totally different diseases (the common cold, hepatitis B, Ebola virus and HIV/AIDS) together under a general diagnosis of *infection*. But think for a moment what it would be like if we did.

Try to imagine the world as it would be if we lumped all those diseases together, the terrible ones and the trivial ones, under the single label of *infection*.

The world of the single disease *infection* would be a scary world indeed. Anyone who developed a sniffle and a runny nose would not be diagnosed with a cold, because in this imaginary world we do not have that word to use as a diagnosis. Instead, they would be told that they have come down with "infection."

Infection! Like those infection outbreaks that happened in Africa and India and killed all those people! The patient would panic and worry that the *infection* might next appear in the liver, or the blood system, or the immune system, or maybe all of them! Perhaps this episode of runny nose and sniffles is the beginning of one of *those* types of *infections*—the ones that overwhelm you and pose a serious risk to health or life!

The analogy is apt, even though I've made it sound a little ridiculous. When you lump different diseases together and you include diseases of greatly different behaviors under the same label, you increase the fear and the dread that the label brings with it.

This is what has happened with the cancers. By constantly referring to this large group of different diseases under the generic title of *cancer* we generate—even if it is only in the subconscious—a deep-seated fear and dread, and create a subtle premonition that somehow any of these two hundred different diseases, even a highly curable one, might mysteriously turn into one of the more aggressive ones.

By attaching the label of *cancer* to all those different diseases you subtly link them all together. The *real* problem is that by linking them together and lumping them under one label, you *remove the predictabil-*

ity of the individual diseases and you create the myth of a single, unpredictable and changeable super-disease which can mysteriously leap from one type of disease to another. I'm now going to show you that cancer is a process, in the same way that "infection" and "inflammation" and "degeneration" are processes, not diseases in themselves.

Our reaction to a diagnosis of a cold or the flu would be fear and dread if we thought that the prognosis might actually be serious, because "everyone knows that infection can affect the liver/blood/immune system next." Lumping together all those conditions that behave so differently into one group would create the myth of a single and totally unpredictable condition. The mere mention of the super-disease *infection* would terrify and paralyze anybody who started getting a cold.

It's the same with the cancers.

When you lump all of the different cancers together as a single mysterious disease that you then call by the one name *cancer*, the predictability of the various different cancers is lost. And there is a tendency to dread *any* of the cancers with the same fear and sense of doom attached to the most serious of them: cancers of the skin seem to be somehow linked to cancer of the pancreas.

When predictability is lost, fear and panic rush in to fill the vacuum.

Now it's not quite as cut-and-dried with the cancers as it is with most of the infectious diseases. Each of the cancers does carry with it some unpredictability—although it is usually pretty limited. Although most cancers are not *totally* predictable, there are well-known limits to that unpredictability. We cannot predict everything, but that doesn't mean that we can't predict anything! You will see in the companion volume, *What You Really Need to Know About Cancer*, how we can predict the future, as far as possible, with each separate cancer, and which factors are important in each disease in predicting its behavior and the chance it will spread. So maybe the comparison with infections is fair after all. We know that a cold won't last six months, but we can't predict whether it will be gone in five days or ten days.

So, having established that all two hundred (or more) cancers do share a common process, let's start by taking a look at that process itself.

The Cancer Process

Cancer is what happens when a group of normal cells start to grow in a disorderly and uncontrollable way and may spread into neighboring areas or to distant parts of the body. In fact, the cancer process consists of three stages.

FIRST, A PARTICULAR GROUP OF CELLS, FOR EXAMPLE IN A DUCT IN A BREAST, STARTS GROWING IN A WAY THAT WE CAN SEE UNDER THE MICROSCOPE IS DISORDERLY AND UNCONTROLLABLE. The cells don't line up in the normal way, their nuclei look peculiar, and their whole appearance—to the expert pathologist—suggests that the cells have escaped from the normal mechanisms that regulate and control cell growth.

SECOND, THE GROWING CELLS INVADE INTO NEIGHBORING AREAS. In normal tissues, the boundaries between one type of tissue and the neighboring areas are strictly demarcated and the tissues on each side of the border, as it were, stay in their allotted territory. In cancers, the cancer cells do not respect the normal boundaries and wander across the border.

Now, if every single cancer did *only* these two things—grow uncontrollably and invade locally—cancers would probably pose a very small risk to health and life, and there would be a fairly small number of deaths from the cancers every year. In most types of cancer, the primary tumor is not the major problem.

THE PROBLEM WITH MOST OF THE COMMON CANCERS IS THAT THEY MAY ALSO DISPLAY A THIRD KIND OF BEHAVIOR: they may spread to distant areas of the body. That process is called *metastasizing*. When a cancer does that, the secondary cancers that it creates in distant areas of the body—for example, the liver or the lungs—are called *metastases*, or *secondaries*. It is the metastases that are most often the real problem and that usually pose a more serious threat to health and life. (There are a relatively small number of situations in which the primary cancer in itself can cause serious illness or death. It can happen, but it's rare.)

So, the process of metastasizing is extremely important and has been the focus of major research efforts over the last fifty years. We now believe that some cancer cells have a high tendency to metastasize, while others do not. We now know a few of the characteristics of highly metastatic cells—the hallmarks, as it were, of aggressive and spreading tendencies.

In many cancers, the pathologist can tell us, to some extent, whether the chance of its spreading to distant areas is high or low or average. At the moment, however, we cannot predict whether an *individual* cancer in a specific person will or will not spread. We can say, for example, that some breast cancers have a high chance of metastasizing. But we cannot tell Mrs. Brown if *hers* will metastasize or not.

And that's a very important point. Because *if* we knew for certain that Mrs. Brown's breast cancer *was not* going to spread, then we would not need to recommend any treatment after surgery in her case. And, if we knew for certain that Mr. Smith's cancer of the bowel *was* going to spread, then we would recommend further treatment after surgery. And if, over the course a few years, Mr. Smith did not develop metastases then we could say for certain that our treatment had worked.

Sadly, we are not there yet. At present we can confidently predict only the *range* of probability of metastasizing, and then recommend treatment options to decrease the risk.

Take breast cancer as an example. If a woman has a small breast cancer (say a centimeter or so) and if it has spread to, let's say, only one of the lymph nodes in the armpit, and if tests on the cancer show that it is likely to respond to hormone treatment, then we can make some pretty good predictions about its behavior and the size of the risk to the patient.

In this case, we can say that for an average type of cancer with these characteristics, the chance of it spreading to distant areas of the body is not high. In fact, the chance of dying of a breast cancer like that over the next ten years, if the patient doesn't take any treatment after the surgery, is about 15 percent. But if the patient does takes hormone tablets for five years after the surgery, that chance is reduced by about one-third, to about 10 percent or so. Of course even a 10 percent chance of the cancer coming back is not trivial—but compared to the general perception of the situation with breast cancer, it is (to most people) surprisingly low.

This is relatively easy to understand. What's difficult to realize, often, is that nobody knows what will happen *in any individual case*. We know the general risks, but not the specific outcome

So nobody can say, whether or not an individual cancer will spread. And therefore nobody can say—*in any individual case*—whether the treatment is preventing recurrence or whether the cancer would not have recurred anyway.

Presently, then, in the majority of cases where we recommend treatment after surgery (as we shall discuss further in Step Three, page 48) we can only talk about the *likelihood* of the cancer spreading and the *likelihood* of the recommended treatment preventing that spread. It's not a very good basis on which to make recommendations, but for the moment it's the best we have.

In the future, we may be able to "fingerprint" the cancer cells much more accurately and perhaps distinguish with certainty those cancers that will not spread from those that will. When we reach that stage, the whole basis on which we recommend treatment will be much more rational and intelligible. And we may see that stage, for some cancers, in the next five or ten years.

So, it's this third step of the cancer process—by which the cancer can spread to distant parts of the body—that represents most of the threat to health and life.

To put it simply then, the cancers are a group of diseases that all share the characteristics of growing in a disorderly and uncontrollable way and potentially spreading to other areas of the body. If you can keep this fundamental principle in mind, then much of the next section, in which we discuss the six steps in coping with a cancer diagnosis, will make a lot of sense.

STEP ONE
"Are You Really Sure It's Cancer, Doctor?"
The Diagnosis

The actual diagnosis is always a shock.

Furthermore, it quite often happens that the initial diagnosis may be *preliminary* and may not be definitive or absolutely certain. In those situations, the uncertainty almost always makes things more difficult for you, as well as for the people around you who want to know what's going on and what's going to be done for you. It's almost always harder for everyone to cope when nobody knows exactly what needs to be coped with.

So this section explains what the diagnosis depends on: when it is likely to be definitive and when it isn't, and what types of further tests may be important.

There are basically only three main ways in which a cancer can be detected and diagnosed. Naturally, this is going to be a considerable oversimplification, but it's helpful to discuss the process of diagnosis under these three broad headings because it will make it easier for you to understand what is going on in your own particular case. It is one of those situations where a map of the forest is useful before you go through the catalog of the trees.

The Ways in Which a First Diagnosis Is Made

Although there are literally hundreds of symptoms and tests that may eventually lead to a diagnosis of a cancer, for practical purposes we can divide the situations into three broad categories. This way of thinking about the process of diagnosis may actually make it easier for you to keep track of where you are at the moment, and what your future options are, as you move along what may feel like a very convoluted and slippery path.

In broad terms, then, the main routes to a diagnosis of a cancer are:

FIRST, DIAGNOSIS FROM A TEST INVESTIGATING A SYMPTOM OR PROBLEM (OR SEVERAL SYMPTOMS OR PROBLEMS) THAT YOU HAVE BEEN EXPERIENCING. A symptom is something you notice yourself, such as a lump in your breast, or chest pain, or blood in your sputum or on your stool. You go to your doctor, who orders a test, or several tests.

If, in your case, a test has led to a *biopsy*—taking a piece or specimen of tissue—then you'll probably want to go straight to page 33, which explains what a biopsy tells us.

If you've had a test or tests, but haven't yet had a biopsy, then you may want to go to page 35, which will discuss the different degrees of certainty and suspicion that nearly all tests will yield.

SECOND, DIAGNOSIS VIA A SCREENING TEST THAT YIELDS AN ABNORMAL RESULT. Screening tests are, by definition, tests done on people who do not have any symptoms or problems related to the disease for which they're being tested. Tests that are used in this way—for screening of people without symptoms—include mammograms, Pap smears, colonoscopies, and prostrate-specific-anitgen (PSA) blood tests. The whole idea of a screening test is to detect the condition—and some cancers are good examples of this—at an early stage when treatment may have a better effect than if it is given later when symptoms have developed.

So, for example, all women who have ever been sexually active should have a regular Pap smear, everybody over the age of fifty should have a rectal examination and probably a colonoscopy, and women should have annual mammograms starting at age fifty. These tests, which have been studied and researched, increase the chance of a cancer being detected at an early stage before it causes symptoms. In these particular cancers, and in some others, the studies show that by detecting the cancers at earlier stages, treatment results are improved and some lives are saved.

That is the idea. And it's a great idea. And it works extremely well in many medical conditions, including quite a few cancers. But there are some problems with every screening test, and it is worth going over them here because you might, at this moment, be hovering near the phone, worrying about the results of a screening test. Or you might have been told that a screening test result is abnormal or uncertain, and you might wonder why screening tests are ever done in the first place if the results don't tell you whether you've got a cancer or not.

Most of the time screening tests give clear and dependable results. But sometimes the results may be unclear or worrying. So let's go back and explain why.

Here's the bottom line: all screening tests sometimes yield unclear results (the correct term is *equivocal*) because there are virtually no tests that have an infallible 100 percent success and reliability record. All biological populations vary. There is a range of every aspect of human life—a range of heights, of intelligence, of athletic prowess, and so on. This goes for most diseases too: there are very many situations in which one cannot be certain whether a particular result is normal or abnormal.

As well as test results sometimes being equivocal, they can also sometimes be wrong—telling you that there is a disease when there isn't, or telling you that there isn't a disease when there is. This means that with every screening test, some people may be very disappointed that there is not a clear result, some may be unduly alarmed, and a few may be falsely reassured. Unpleasant, but inevitable. At present, we don't have the technology to eradicate those uncertain and unsettling results even though there are very few of them.

THIRD, DIAGNOSIS AS AN INCIDENTAL FINDING DURING A PROCEDURE FOR SOMETHING ELSE. It sometimes happens, and it is not all that rare, that a procedure is carried out for a purpose not related to a cancer (or even the suspicion of a cancer) but during the procedure a cancer is found. You may be having a hysterectomy for fibroids, for example, when evidence of a cancer is found.

If this happened to you—an unexpected incidental finding during a procedure for something else—then psychologically it is very tough indeed (as you may be feeling right now).

But take heart. It is usually a good thing if a cancer is discovered as an incidental finding. Generally speaking, cancers that do not cause you any problems or symptoms usually have a somewhat better prognosis than those that call attention to themselves by producing symptoms or problems.

However, the lack of symptoms often makes the intellectual shock worse. Almost every patient to whom this happens says, "But I was feeling so well." And they mean it. If you are feeling unwell, you may be prepared psychologically for a diagnosis of something potentially serious. But if you have no problems, much less a suspicion of a cancer, the shock is often much greater.

The secret to coping with that shock—in line with the central message of this book—is to get informed. It's worth spending a little time trying to get an overview of your cancer. As I pointed out earlier, a few cancers pose an immediate (and sometimes serious) threat to you, but most cancers do not. So it's really important that you try to get a handle on what has been discovered in your case. That information—the map of the forest—will greatly help you in marshaling your own coping strategies. So, even though a diagnosis out of the blue may well knock you sharply off balance, you can help yourself steadily to regain that balance by finding out what kind of a problem you are now dealing with.

A Brief Guide To the Tissue Diagnosis

In most cases, one of the three routes that we've just described will lead to your clinical team organizing a biopsy, a sample of the suspicious tissue or portion of the organ in which the abnormality has been detected. Biopsies are relatively straightforward.

The word *biopsy* simply means taking a piece of tissue. There are many dozens of ways in which that can be done, and a lot depends on the part of the body in which the problem is situated. For example if there is a lump in the breast a biopsy can be taken with a thin needle after a little local anesthetic. The procedure is quite minor and takes only a few minutes. On the other hand, a biopsy from a problem area in the brain is considerably more complex. It requires a proper operation with a general anesthetic and may take an hour or longer.

In the case of many of the organs inside the abdomen, a biopsy can be taken during a laparoscopy. Usually done under general anesthetic this procedure does not require a full incision and involves only inserting a thin telescope through the abdominal wall, by which a biopsy can be taken. There are different ways of doing the same thing depending on the part of the body involved. For instance, during a *bronchoscopy*, the surgeon will examine your lungs and bronchial tree with a thin telescope called a *bronchoscope*, then slot fine tweezers into the bronchoscope and take a piece of tissue from the wall of a *bronchus*, one of the tubes that conduct the air into your lungs. During *colonoscopy*, a similar method is used to take a biopsy from your colon (large bowel) or rectum. Similarly, it is possible to look at and take a biopsy from the structure in the middle of the chest, between the lungs and around the heart, called the *mediastinum*. That procedure is called a *mediastinoscopy*.

Depending on the exact site of the suspicious area, sometimes you may need to have a separate operation for the surgeon to get an adequate sample of the area. So you may need to have a *laparotomy* (an operation in which the abdomen is opened) or a *thoracotomy* (opening the chest to allow access to the lungs or the heart or the mediastinum) or, in the case of the suspicion of a brain tumor, a *craniotomy* (opening of a part of the skull to allow access to an area of the brain).

In some areas, sufficient information can be obtained from the suspicious area or lesion by using a thin needle and taking a thin core of the tissue. This is called a *needle biopsy*. Using an even finer needle and sucking out some cells from the tumor is called a *fine needle aspirate* and may, in some circumstances, give enough information to plan further tests, including a larger biopsy. (There is a good diagram of these procedures in *What You Really Need to Know About Cancer.*)

The *bone marrow* is in some ways a special case. The bone marrow is where the cells in the bloodstream are produced. When there are malignant cells in the bloodstream, as occurs in the various types of leukemia and some other conditions, a bone marrow sample is taken. Sometimes this consists of inserting a fine needle into the bone marrow inside the pelvis. The needle goes in—under anesthetic, of course—near the top inside part of the buttock area and a sample of the cells is sucked out. In other circumstances, an actual piece of bone marrow, including the inner surface of the bone, may be needed. This involves basically the same type of procedure but with a slightly different needle. In any event, you can think of these bone marrow tests as, basically, biopsies of the blood-making site.

What a Tissue Diagnosis Means

In the great majority of cases—and there are a very small number of exceptions—the whole plan of treatment and the discussions about your condition and your plans, is based on the pathologist's examination of the biopsy under the microscope. That is what is meant by the phrase *tissue diagnosis*, having the actual cancer cells under the microscope. Broadly speaking, there are four main clinical settings possible with the biopsy.

FIRST, A BIOPSY HAS BEEN TAKEN AND THE RESULT IS CLEAR. This is the most common situation. You have had a lump in the breast. Or a bronchoscopy was done to investigate a shadow on your chest X-ray and an abnormality was found. The pathologist will examine a piece of the abnormal area. In most situations this process takes a few days. Remember, now, what I've said before about the way cancers behave and the rate at which they change. Although a few days may feel like a very long time, it is of enormous importance that the tissue sample be carefully examined, and it is genuinely worthwhile taking the necessary amount of time to ensure the result is trustworthy. As one of my patients said about the expertise of the pathologist, "You need a really good map-reader in order to trust the 'You Are Here' sticker."

In the majority of situations, the result of the biopsy is conclusive. The pathologist's report analyses literally dozens of different features of the cells and can state with certainty whether or not there are cancer cells present and, if there are, the way they are arranged. The pathologist analyzes many features about the cells' appearance, important features that have been shown partly to predict how the cancer is going to behave.

The most important of those features are usually:

The *type* of the cancer, meaning which tissue it started in. This is important because, for example, cancer of the breast that has spread to the lung still behaves like cancer of the breast and is sensitive to the kind of treatment used for cancer of the breast.

The *size* of the cancer, and—for some kinds of cancer, for example, the bowel and the uterus—how deep into the surrounding normal tissue it invades.

The *grade* of the cancer, meaning how aggressive it looks under the microscope. The way a cancer is graded varies from site to site. Pathologists all over the world look at certain standard features of the cancer cells and can correlate these with the way the cancer behaves, as a result of large numbers of research studies looking at those features and the outcomes. Some features are common to most cancers—for example, very big nuclei occupying most of the cell, and many cells being seen in the process of reproducing. But some features are specific to a specific cancer cell. So the grading system for cancer of the breast, say, is similar to, but not the same as brain tumors.

Usually, the pathologist can also determine much more than that. She or he can take slides of the tumor and stain them with different antibodies that bind to different kinds of molecular patterns on the cancer cells. For example, special stains can be used on breast cancer to see if there are estrogen or progesterone receptors on the cells, or an antigen (molecule) called *her2/neu* which makes the cancer cells susceptible to the drug Herceptin (trastuzumab). (See Table 1, The Features of a Cancer that the Pathologist Assesses, page 237; and Table 2, Special Stains that Can Be Done on some Cancers, page 241.)

What You Really Need to Know About Cancer shows how these factors (and others that the pathologist notes and includes in the report) are important in determining the likely behavior of the cancer in future, and the best treatment options.

With most biopsies, then, the pathologist can determine clearly what type of cancer is present and how aggressive, or what grade, it is. Sometimes, however, the result isn't clear, and when that happens it's very upsetting to you and your family. So let's take some time to discuss what "We don't have the full answer yet" actually means. This brings us to the second clinical setting after a biopsy.

SECOND, A BIOPSY HAS BEEN TAKEN BUT THE RESULT IS NOT CLEAR. "You've got the piece of abnormal tissue right there under the microscope. Why can't you tell what it is?" When you first think about it, it might seem that a biopsy should always yield a definite and certain answer. But there are several situations in which a definitive answer isn't clear. Think of analyzing handwriting. If the sample of the writing includes a variety of letters and flourishes, the analyst may well be able to identify the writer. But if the sample is only a fragment, it becomes increasingly difficult.

It's worth considering a couple of examples, because this result, naturally enough, causes so much distress.

There are some cancers that under the microscope appear to be so dormant and slow growing that it is actually difficult to determine whether they are truly cancers or not. One example is borderline tumor of the ovary.

In other cases, the cancer cells may have lost so many of the features of the cells from which they originated that it is not possible to say with certainty where the tumor started. In fact between 5 and 10 percent of all cancers fit into this category and some are known as *cancers of unknown primary*—it can be seen that the cancer cells form little gland-like formations or have other features, but have lost all of the identifying features of the tissue that they started from (e.g., lung, bowel or breast). It's important that you know about that, because many people, when they hear the diagnosis of unknown primary, think that this simply means the pathologist is not very good.

In an increasing number of cases these days, much more information can be gained by using special stains. If the cells have estrogen receptors, for example, it is quite likely that the cancer originated from the breast.

THIRD, A BIOPSY HAS NOT YET BEEN TAKEN AND THE DIAGNOSIS IS BASED ON THE RESULT OF A TEST. If one of the tests that you had suggests a cancer diagnosis but a biopsy has not yet been done, then this period of waiting is naturally going to be filled with anxiety. It can hardly be otherwise. As one patient put it, "It's the feeling of not having anything to go on that knots you up. You almost long for news, whether it's good or bad, because it's better to know than not know."

Almost everybody can understand those types of feelings. If you don't know whether there is something serious going on or not, then you don't know how to prepare yourself, or even what to prepare yourself for. You are genuinely in a kind of limbo.

There are only two questions that may help you get things into perspective.

The first is how strongly did the test result—the X-ray or scan or blood test—suggest a cancer diagnosis?

The second is when is the next step—the biopsy or other test—being done?

If you can focus on the answers to these two questions, you may be better able to cope with those queasy feelings of uncertainty that will probably creep up on you from time to time.

It is better to focus on the day-to-day events at this stage, than to start worrying, or researching, or surfing the Net about the way in which the cancer would be treated, *if* that's the diagnosis. If you are mired in uncertainty—and everyone knows how very unpleasant that is—then you'll be better off acknowledging that uncertainty than driving yourself crazy by drawing up plans for each eventuality. Of course waiting is a really uncomfortable experience, but if you can see that for yourself and can acknowledge how uncomfortable it makes you feel, you can, to some extent, contain the anxiety, and at least draw a line around it. Acknowledging uncertainty usually helps your coping strategies. Denying the feeling usually doesn't.

FOURTH, A BIOPSY CANNOT BE TAKEN. There are a very few areas of the body where the process of taking a sample of tissue is so hazardous that a biopsy can't be done safely. Although this situation is rare, it does apply, for example, to certain crucial areas of the brain, particularly the brainstem, which is the stalk-like back part of the brain and forms the major highway controlling and conducting almost all information from the body to the brain. Injuries to the brainstem would be so devastating that most types of biopsy are too hazardous. If there is a suspicious lesion in that area, it will usually be treated as if it were a brain tumor, even without a tissue diagnosis. There are a few other situations like that, but they are rare. In these uncommon situations, often the treatment plan has to be based on imaging—CT or MRI or some other scan—without a tissue diagnosis.

What Next?
It will help you to know how your medical team is planning to make the definitive diagnosis if there isn't one yet. So, it will be of real help to you to know if there's going to be another biopsy, and if so when, or if special stains are being used on the tissue sample, or more blood tests are being done, or if the tumor sample—as is commonly done—is being shown to other pathologists or sent to other centers. These are

relatively simple questions to ask, and to answer, and knowing the plan for the next stage will make you feel a bit easier.

The Two Questions That Are Most Commonly Asked

This may be the appropriate time to deal with two questions which go through most people's minds at the time of a diagnosis. I'm including them here to reassure you that, however embarrassed or perplexed you may feel about these two issues, you are not alone. Many people—patients and friends—feel uncertain about them.

THE FIRST QUESTION: *Is the diagnosis in my case* certain *or* suspicious?

At first, this point may seem obvious, but for many people it does need some thought.

Whenever we hear the word *cancer* from a physician or health care professional, we immediately feel that, as one patient put it, "The jury is back and the verdict is final."

Now sometimes the diagnosis is certain. Although, as this entire book points out, the outlook for the future depends not on the word *cancer* alone, but on which *kind* of cancer, at what *stage*, and what kind of *treatment options* are possible.

So always take a mental breath and ask this first question: is the diagnosis *certain* or *suspicious*? Sometimes you're not absolutely sure what your doctor said—or meant—and it may take some thought and some questions to your medical team to find out whether the diagnosis is a preliminary suspicion or a certain and definitive one.

This is probably hard for you. Even so, it's worth thinking about the issues that we've discussed in Step One so far, and then asking your doctor or other member of the medical team where they are in your particular case. Understanding something about the uncertainties will make it easier for you to comprehend the answers that you hear.

THE SECOND QUESTION: *Why couldn't this have been found earlier?*

Hindsight—as the saying goes—is 20/20.

It is not unusual to look back on any major event and to ask ourselves why it happened, and what we could have done differently that would have made things turn out differently. This is a normal reaction. It's the "if only" reaction, and it is a response that is so common that it is almost universal.

When the diagnosis is one of the cancers, the "if only" response is even more intense—partly because of the universal sense of dread and fear attached to the word *cancer*. The deeper the fear, the more persistent the feeling that it could have been avoided.

There are three aspects of the way cancers develop that may partly account for (and so help you to understand) the apparent lateness of the diagnosis. Those three factors are: the location of the cancer (where it starts), the speed (or slowness) with which cancers grow, and how common the symptoms are. Let's deal with each of those three aspects in some detail.

FIRST, WHERE THE PROBLEM STARTS. In many areas of the body, a group of cells growing in a disorderly and uncontrollable way will produce a symptom that you notice yourself. The amount of growth that can occur *before you notice it* depends on where exactly in your body the process starts. In some areas of the body, you'll notice a problem soon after it starts, in other areas it may take a longer time.

For example, you are likely to notice a change in the skin on your face at a very early stage. The skin is quite tight and there is not a great deal of tissue underneath it, and also we look at our faces regularly. That means that skin cancers on the face (either the common and relatively docile ones—the basal cell cancers or the squamous cancers—or the potentially more aggressive and rare ones—the melanomas) are likely to be detected early. But the same kind of problem somewhere

where the skin is looser and not often examined—in the middle of your back, for example, or on the back of your calf or your sole—may grow for a longer time before it is noticed. This is a simple example of how the place (the location), of a problem, inside the body or out, can make a difference to the immediacy of the detection.

Another example is the breast, where a lump is relatively easy to detect by routine mammography because the breast tissue is relatively accessible to X-rays. And mammography, which, as almost every woman will point out, is not necessarily comfortable for the patient, but is, technically, fairly easy to perform.

The breast, then, is relatively accessible to X-rays. But the ovaries, located in the pelvis, are not. The female pelvis is a brilliant piece of evolutionary design for ensuring the protection of a growing fetus during pregnancy. The uterus and the ovaries are soundly protected by the rigid cage of bone, which ensures the safety of a pregnancy, but also makes them relatively inaccessible. So, the down side of the design of the pelvis is that pelvic organs are relatively protected from signaling early signs of trouble. If a mass begins to develop on an ovary, it will not cause symptoms that the woman will notice for a long time (unlike a breast lump) and, for that reason, cancer of the ovary will have spread around the abdomen in about two-thirds of cases before it is diagnosed.

Hence the position in the body—the geographical location of the tumor—drastically affects the ease or difficulty of an early diagnosis.

SECOND, THE SLOWNESS OF CANCER GROWTH. Contrary to what most people believe, the vast majority of cancers actually grow fairly slowly. In fact, the average cancer cell probably divides into two cells about once a month. There are certain tumors where the multiplication speed is faster than that, particularly in the childhood cancers, and there are a few tumors that are much slower, but that's a reasonable average. (In fact, this topic is so important that I've devoted extensive space to it, with a very helpful illustration, in *What You Really Need to Know About Cancer.*)

The bottom line is significant. Imagine a group of cells dividing every month (that's not exactly how it happens, but it's a useful analogy). After a year, one cell will have produced approximately four thousand cells. At that rate of multiplication, it will take two and a half years for the mass of cells to reach the size of a small grape, about one billion cells. In other words, even if we could detect every tumor when it was grape-sized, the tumor would still have had two and a half years of reproduction before we found it. So most cancers do not, in fact, grow very fast.

This reality is very different from what most people think—and is another unfortunate result of lumping all two hundred or so cancers together under a single label. From reports in the media most people get the impression that every case of cancer is an emergency. Now impression is also (in part) the result of the way we give priority to patients receiving treatment for cancer. Many types of treatment need a very exact time schedule. Chemotherapy and radiation, for example, must both be given on an exact schedule. Missing some days or doses is hazardous both in terms of loss of efficacy and in terms of possible side effects. Now while this, quite appropriately, means that cancer patients receiving treatment must get priority, it does not mean that *the cancer itself* is an emergency, although most people assume it is.

The result is that it becomes almost conventional wisdom to imagine that all cases of cancer will cause serious medical problems in a very short time, and that once a cancer begins, it will cause noticeable or detectable problems in a few days or weeks.

In the vast majority of cases—and it is worth stressing this point again—the situation is nothing like this. There are actually very few situations in which a cancer causes problems in so short a time. But the sense of dread and fear is amplified by the sense of urgency that often accompanies it. So in many cases the answer to the question, "Why could it not have been detected earlier?" is related to the time-scale of the cancers themselves, not the failure to do tests often enough.

THIRD, HOW OFTEN DOES THE SAME SYMPTOM OCCUR WHEN THERE IS NOTH-ING SERIOUS GOING ON? As the saying goes, "Headaches are common, brain tumors are rare." Some cancers—in fact, quite a few—may initially cause symptoms that are very common indeed.

This means that it can be very difficult to identify the few cases in which something potentially serious is going on from the very large number of benign cases, where nothing much is happening. That is why symptoms that *might* be associated with a cancer should be checked out by a doctor. This is particularly true for headaches, for example. Your doctor, taking some details of the headaches, may well decide which situations need further tests and which do not. Another example is bleeding during or after a bowel movement. Once again, hemorrhoids are common and colo-rectal cancer is by comparison fairly rare, but if you have bleeding and your doctor does not see any hemorrhoids, then further testing might well be important.

These two examples illustrate how difficult it can be to identify the rare case of a cancer. I am not saying this as an apologist for the medical profession. I simply want to point out that we generally do our best, and that *all* biological problems—including symptoms and cancers—are quite variable.

And as I noted earlier, hindsight is 20/20. Looking back on a problem, you can almost always identify a moment when a symptom began, and it is very tempting to blame yourself for not having gone to the doctor sooner, or to blame the doctor for not having made the correct diagnosis instantly.

As a cancer physician I often see this reaction—it is sometimes called *retrospective guilt*, or even *retrospective blame*.

With a word as scary as *cancer*, people often feel that any period of time that elapses during the process of diagnosis has somehow jeopardized them. In fact, that is very rare. And those feelings are part of the baggage that is brought in with all the reactions to the word *cancer*.

STEP TWO
"Do I Actually Need All These Tests?"
Staging

STEP
TWO

Staging tests are, according to some, "the insult that is added to the injury." Often, they seem to do no more than delay getting the treatment started. But they do matter, and this section explains why.

In particular, the way the treatment for a cancer is planned often depends largely on the stage it has reached. Early stages are frequently treated differently from later stages.

This section will help you to understand why staging tests, although they seem to be a nuisance and an irritation, really do matter.

The Principles of Staging Tests
One patient compared staging tests to "a patrol of the premises by security guards—they usually don't find anything, but they know how to sound the alert if there's trouble."

The point is that some cancers can invade to a greater extent locally than is apparent when the doctor examines you, and some can spread to distant areas of the body without causing any symptoms or noticeable trouble. If either of these things has happened, the treatment plan will have to be modified accordingly. So the screening tests are done in order to find out if there is anything unexpected going on. And that means that a very large number of people will be having tests which turn out *not* to show anything unexpected. It's a nuisance, but it's important.

The staging tests are selected on two basic and simple principles which we can best express as the answers to these two important questions:

If this particular cancer were to spread, where in the body it is most likely to spread to?

Which tests both have a high likelihood of detecting something wrong at an early stage and do not usually produce a false-alarm or false-positive? That means they don't give the appearance of a serious abnormality when there is actually nothing wrong.

I can best illustrate these two principles with two tests in breast cancer—a bone scan, and a blood test called the *carcino embryonic antigen* (CEA).

The bone scan is actually quite a useful—and subtle—test. A small dose of a harmless radioactive isotope called *technetium* is given to you by intravenous injection. When the technetium circulates in the body, it is taken up almost exclusively by the cells in the bone that actually make the bone tissue. These cells are called *osteoblasts*, and where they take up the isotope the bone scan will show a fine pattern of tiny black dots.

Now, in many cancers, the cancer cells settle in the bone and start destroying the bits of bone around them. This provokes a reaction by the defence team, the osteoblasts.

This reaction is almost always provoked if a group of breast cancer cells lodges in the bone. With other cancers, that reaction doesn't always happen. But with breast cancer if there is even a relatively small group of cancer cells spreading to and settling in a bone—such as the spine, or the long bones of the arms or legs—the bone scan is highly likely to show them as a larger than average black splodge, or *hot spot* as it is called.

Now it also happens that other problems—particularly in the joints, such as arthritis—can also produce hot spots on the bone scan, but arthritis and most noncancerous problems usually look different (and appear in different patterns and place) from cancer metastases. So in the great majority of cases, an experienced radiologist can look at the bone scan and state with considerable certainty whether there any areas that might be secondaries or not. In some cases, the bone scan itself cannot distinguish between a probably benign appearance such as arthritis and a probably metastatic appearance. Then, X-rays of the area or CT scans of the area will be required.

So even if the patient has no symptoms related to that area—no pain or discomfort—the bone scan will probably pick up an early secondary or metastasis. That's what makes it so useful as a staging test, and that's why it's worth having one, when recommended, even though you may have no symptoms or problems in your bones.

That's how a bone scan works. And because breast cancer has a high predilection for spreading to the bones, in any situation where the breast cancer has demonstrated a higher than average risk of spreading—if the lymph nodes are positive, for example—a bone scan is worth doing.

It's a different story for the carcino embryonic antigen (CEA). CEA is a substance secreted by several different cancer cells, including colorectal, breast, and some lung cancers. In breast cancer, however, the levels of CEA are usually normal when the breast cancer has not spread. The levels rise above normal only when there is a high total amount of cancer. Furthermore, the CEA is often raised in other conditions. In fact, people who smoke heavily can have a high CEA level even when there is nothing wrong with them. So, given the low rate of success in detecting small amounts of metastases, and given also the false-positive rate, the CEA is not worth doing as a staging test.

By and large these two principles are used in deciding which staging tests should be done for each type of cancer after diagnosis.

Which brings us round to the question, "Do I really have to have these tests?" The answer is that having any tests is not compulsory. Nobody's giving you an order. *But* in each type of cancer there is a group of tests that have a fair chance of detecting any unexpected problems. If your particular cancer has a moderate or higher chance of spreading, the fact that your doctor is suggesting you have a bunch of tests of, say, your bones and liver and lungs, does *not* mean that she expects to find problems there. It means that she wishes to prove conclusively that there are no problems there.

So, those irritating staging tests are a sign that your treatment plan is based on sound factual knowledge. (Table 3 on page 242 lists The Most Common Types of Tests and What They Mean.)

STEP
THREE

STEP THREE
"Why Do I Need More Than One Type of Treatment?"
Treatment Types and What They Do

This is going to be a very brief introduction to the principles of the four main types of cancer treatment—surgery, radiotherapy (radiation oncology), chemotherapy, and biological therapy (including hormone therapy).

In this bird's-eye view I'm going to explain in a couple of paragraphs how each of the four types of treatment works. You may find that you know this already but quite often it's easy to be confused about, say, radiotherapy, so Step Three will just set the scene for you.

In Part Two I set out in greater detail what's actually involved in the different types of treatment, plus some of the specific actions and side effects.

As I said in the opening pages of this book, the general concepts and the treatment options are covered here, but if you want to know how *particular* types of cancer—breast, lung, leukemia, and the others—are treated, it's worth reading the relevant section in *What You Really Need to Know About Cancer*, which explains the specific strategies in each.

Treatment: Is There a "Best Kind?"

Treatment plans are often confusing.

The problem is that each of the four types of treatment does a different job—and in some situations you need several types of treatment to deal with different aspects of the cancer.

That fact by itself often causes some confusion.

Some patients are confused about why they need any treatment after surgery, some are confused about why they need, say, two types of therapy (maybe local radiotherapy and chemotherapy), and some patients become worried if they are not being given all four types of treatment and want to know if they are being short-changed ("Am I getting second-class treatment? Does the team know something about my condition that they're not telling me?"). Others may think that they are being *over*-treated and feel that they don't really need all the treatment methods that are being used.

To be honest, it is confusing.

It is also confusing that there isn't a single "best type" of treatment for each site of cancer—for example some cancers of the breast need chemotherapy and radiotherapy, some need hormonal treatment, and so on.

The reason—which won't be a surprise to those of you who have read the earlier parts of this book—is that cancer is not one single disease, and therefore there is no one single treatment. Unlike shower caps, for example, one size does *not* fit all!

As I've said several times, the cancers are a group of two hundred different diseases that may need treatment at many different stages of development. Furthermore, patients are not all the same—some are young, some are old, some have other medical conditions, some don't—and that means that the risks and the side effects of the different treatment methods may be quite different in Mrs. Smith than they are in Mr. Brown.

So all those different factors—the type of cancer, the stage, the age and medical state of the patient—create a large number of different combinations. Hence the best or most appropriate type of treatment will to some extent be individualized to you, and will depend on the tumor and its stage, and your own medical state.

The members of your medical team will match you up with the therapy, or combination of therapies, that offers you the highest chance of success with the lowest chance of side effects. That means that even if you have friends and neighbors with the same diagnosis, they may be receiving different types of treatment from you. If you have cancer of the breast, say, there may be reasons that hormone tablets are not recommended to you, while they are for your neighbor who also has breast cancer.

This section will set out some of the criteria by which these treatment options are recommended.

What's the best kind of cancer treatment? It completely depends on your particular situation. Because there are hundreds of different clinical situations—depending on the type of the cancer, the stage, the part of the body that the tumor is in, and so on—there are hundreds of facts that need to be considered in the selection of treatment for any one person.

In your case, your medical team may recommend one, some, or even all of these treatment methods. That is why it is extremely important that you discuss the individual treatment approach with your medical team.

Surgery

Surgery is the oldest method of treating any type of cancer and there are records of surgical techniques going back many hundreds of years.

The important point to realize here is that *surgery is treatment for the local disease*, that is, the disease in one particular part of the body.

Sometimes that's all that is needed, but sometimes it's not enough. You can help yourself to ask the right kind of question by focusing on the following four topics:

Which area of the body is involved? This largely determines what the surgery is going to be like: if it is going to be a big operation or a small one, and what the effect will be on nearby organs. After surgery in the abdomen, for example, how quickly will bowel function return; in the lungs what will your breathing be like afterwards, and so on?

After the surgery, will additional local therapy be required? In other words, is the chance of the cancer recurring in the same area high, or low, or moderate? If it's moderate or high, often radiotherapy will be recommended to reduce that chance of a local recurrence.

After the surgery, will additional systemic treatment—such as chemotherapy, hormone, or biologic therapy, that reaches all areas of the body—be recommended?

Are there alternatives to surgery or alternatives to big surgery? For example, in prostate cancer, what are the risks and benefits of using radiotherapy instead of surgery? In breast cancer, what are the risks and benefits of using radiotherapy after lumpectomy, compared to the bigger operation, mastectomy, which removes the entire breast?

In thinking about and discussing these topics with your surgical team, remember one important point (often a source of confusion, and even doubt). Whether or not further treatment is required after surgery depends on the *type of cancer* and on the way it is likely to behave, not on the personal skill of your surgeon!

In other words, the need for chemotherapy and/or radiotherapy after surgery does *not* mean that your surgeon didn't succeed or did not do a good job. It means that in your particular case, the cancer itself poses a significant risk of recurring or spreading. It is very common for the surgery to be successful, meaning that all the visible tumor was removed and the phrase "we got it all" is accurate about the local cancer, but there may still be a significant chance of recurrence or spread. For that reason, further therapy may be recommended after surgery.

This occurs often, and there can be some confusion on the patient's part about whether the right operation was done or was performed properly. Hopefully what I am saying here will clear up that common sense of confusion!

Radiotherapy (Radiation Oncology)

Radiotherapy is treatment in which an area of the body is given a high dose of radiation—rays that are similar in some respects to X-rays but different in that they are produced with the intention of damaging any growing cells in the area exposed to them.

These rays are usually created in specific machines called *linear accelerators* and are very closely controlled and monitored by highly specialized systems. There are some diagrams of what the machines look like and how the rays penetrate the skin in *What You Really Need to Know About Cancer.*

It is important to realize that radiation, like surgery, is a *local treatment*. In other words, it treats the area that gets the radiation only, and has little or no effect on any cancer cells outside the area being treated. Although many people know this, it can still be confusing, and some patients are really perplexed when it is recommended that they have radiotherapy after their chemotherapy, for example after a lumpectomy for breast cancer.

The single most important feature of radiotherapy is that the radiation passes through normal structures—such as the skin or lungs or bowel or spinal cord, depending on the area of the body involved.

Nowadays it is possible to "focus" the radiation very precisely in the cancer area, and to reduce the damage to normal structures in front or behind that area. There are several ways to do this:

By using several different directions (or fields), each of which is concentrated on the cancer, but each of which affects different areas (say, of the skin or bowel).

By using radiation that has the appropriate properties for a particular cancer—for example, radiation that gives out much of its energy near the skin surface and doesn't penetrate very far is good for superficial cancers, whereas radiation that gives most of its energy deep in the tissues does less damage to the skin.

And finally, by using tailor-made radiation fields that are "trimmed" to include all of the tumor mass and very little of the surrounding normal tissues.

Obviously, the planning of radiation treatment is a major and important procedure. Nowadays, the actual imaging of the cancer area can be done with greater and greater accuracy. Although it's a tricky and somewhat exacting process—and probably quite boring for you!—it's crucially important because it drastically affects how much damage can be done to the cancer cells while avoiding the normal cells in the area.

Chemotherapy

Chemotherapy involves the treatment of cancers by drugs that, to some extent, damage all growing cells. Chemotherapy drugs work in the treatment of the cancers because, overall they do much more damage to cancer cells than they do to normal cells.

A cancer mass has many more growing cells inside it than normal tissue does, and that is why chemotherapy agents generally do more extensive damage to cancers than they do to normal tissues.

However, by their very nature most chemotherapy agents do some damage to all growing cells. That is why many of them cause your hair to fall out (temporarily), because they damage the growing cells at the hair root. Similarly, they may cause mouth sores by damaging the growing cells in the mouth. More importantly, they can affect the growing cells in the bone marrow, which are responsible for making the various components of blood. Hence, many (but not all) chemotherapy agents can reduce your white cells count (a condition called *neutropenia*) making you more susceptible to infections and fevers. They can also reduce your platelets (a condition caused *thrombocytopenia*) which are important in helping blood to clot. Hence you may develop bruises or bleeding. Chemotherapy can also affect the red cells (causing anemia) that contain hemoglobin and this would cause you to look pale and to feel tired and short of breath.

Most chemotherapy agents also cause some nausea and vomiting, and although this is a common side effect of most of the drugs, it isn't directly related to their ability to damage growing cells. In fact it appears that there are certain centers in the brain which are particularly sensitive to certain types of chemicals in the bloodstream. These centers are called the chemotactic trigger zone (CTZ) and the vomiting center (VC).

Biological Therapy (Including Hormone Therapy)

Whereas chemotherapy agents are basically drugs that damage all growing cells (to a greater or lesser extent), biologic agents are drugs (usually complex manufactured proteins) that seek and bind to specific targets on the surface of cancer cells. They are—to use a crude analogy—like "smart bombs" that "home in" on specific characteristics of the cancer cells and, hopefully, avoid doing damage to normal cells, which do not have those targets on their surface. When they work well, biologic agents produce much less "collateral damage."

The earliest drugs that worked by biological means, specifically targeting cancer cells by altering one aspect of the internal environment, were hormone treatments, which are still today a major part of the treatment of some cancers, notably cancer of the prostate and cancer of the breast.

Later I'll show you how biological and hormone treatments are both evolving. Here, the most important thing to realize is that not all cancers can be treated by hormone or biological treatments. There are hormone agents or biologic agents presently available for a lot of cancers, but not for all. For example, if you have breast cancer and it happens to have estrogen receptors on it, then hormone treatments (such as tamoxifen or letrozole) can be used. If it doesn't have estrogen receptors, then those treatments will not be effective. If the cancer cells happen to have a marker called *her2/neu* on them (see page 67) then a drug called trastuzumab (Herceptin) can be used in addition to chemotherapy. But if the cancer cells do not have that marker on them, Herceptin will not be of any value.

These are just a couple of examples. Biological therapy is evolving very rapidly indeed, and new biologic agents are coming available for use in different tumors all the time. So you and your medical team will need to discuss those new agents as they emerge.

Treatment Options–When Can You Choose?

In some cancer situations, there are several approaches to the treatment, and all of them are basically equivalent. When that happens, then you can choose among them.

In other situations, there is only one approach that is known to be effective, or at least more effective than anything else. In those situations, you have to decide whether or not the recommended plan is actually acceptable to you.

Where there are several options, all equivalent, your own preferences are highly relevant. Here's an example. In certain cases of breast cancer we know that after removing the breast (mastectomy), radiotherapy is usually *not* required: there is no additional benefit in adding radiotherapy in most cases. On the other hand, there are also many cases in which the surgery is more limited—using lumpectomy or its equivalent, instead of removing the entire breast. In these latter cases, studies show very clearly that radiotherapy given after the operation *is* required. Without radiotherapy after limited surgery, the incidence of local recurrence, the cancer coming back in the breast or in the scar, is significant. With it, the chance of local recurrence is markedly reduced. It's not zero, but it's much lower than it would otherwise have been.

So, for most cases of breast cancer where the tumor is not very large, we could say that limited surgery plus radiotherapy is the same as mastectomy, in terms of local treatment. In other words, they both achieve the same result in minimizing the chance of the cancer coming back in the breast area or near the scar.

This is where your preferences are paramount.

You might, let's say, live a long way from the nearest radiotherapy center, or it might be very awkward for you to come in to the center every day. You might also feel that the final cosmetic result is not of major importance. If so, then you might choose (as many people do) to have a "once only" mastectomy, which does not require radiotherapy afterwards.

If, on the other hand, you feel that the final cosmetic result is important and you don't mind the extra time and inconvenience of get-ting the radiotherapy, and you can accept the slightly increased chance of local recurrence, then you might choose to have lumpectomy with radiotherapy as the local treatment, instead of mastectomy.

The bottom line is simply this: which treatment or combination of treatment has the highest success rate in treating this particular cancer in this particular situation?

If there are two or more combinations of treatment that have equal success rates, then it is usual to select the combination that has the lowest incidence of side effects and long-term consequences.

STEP FOUR
"Do I Have to Have Treatment Now?"
Taking a Breath–and a Moment to Assess the Situation and the Future

Another problem with thinking of all the cancers as one single rapidly progressive disease is that it's very difficult to think calmly about treatment options and make decisions.

If you think of cancer as a single, universally and rapidly fatal disease—which, unfortunately, the majority of people still do—then you may feel a strong urge to start treatment as quickly as possible. Furthermore, if you think of every type of cancer as posing an immediate and serious threat to health and life, you might also tend to play down or even dismiss the severity or consequences of any side effects of treatment because you feel that the ends justify the means. While that is certainly true in some situations, it is not true in others.

This section will help you appreciate the range of treatment options by matching them, as far as possible, to the degree of risk in your own case.

This section is all about taking a breath—and spending a moment or two discussing and thinking about the situation, and about the options for treatment which may improve it.

For most people, the news of the diagnosis is truly shocking. And the shock is made worse, as I've pointed out repeatedly, if you believe that all the cancers are one single disease requiring urgent and immediate treatment.

That's why I want to make the point in this section that what really matters is balancing the benefits and the risks of the *particular* treatment options in *your particular* case.

There is no universal rule that if it's cancer it's got to be treated *today*, no matter how toxic the treatment.

What matters is getting a true and accurate picture of your own situation from your medical team, and matching the treatment with the risk.

As you will see here, there are some situations where treatment can, and should, be delayed. There are many others where it shouldn't. And there are a few where there needs to be considerable discussion before treatment decisions can be made.

So take a leisurely look at this section. I hope that it will inform you and supply you with a background understanding of the situation, so that when you talk to your medical team, you can focus on the details of your own particular case.

Balancing Potential Benefits Against Potential Risks

This question bothers almost every person who has a cancer diagnosis: "Do I actually need treatment now?" (Or, more commonly, "Do I actually need *more* treatment now, after the initial surgery or the biopsy?")

Because there are so many different cancers, and because each of them can be diagnosed at various stages in various people, it's actually quite difficult to arrange the spectrum of treatment options into a sensible all-embracing scheme. Nevertheless, I am going to try to do that now. I will lay out a seven-category system that groups the various cancer situations together based on the primary objective or aim of treatment.

This approach is actually novel, so it might seem to that I am putting very different tumors together under the same heading.

In a way, that's exactly what I am doing. And it may be very useful to you.

It may actually help you to understand the whole objective of the treatment of your own particular tumor if you see it compared with the treatment of another tumor. It is often easier to understand a plan of treatment when you see a range of different situations in which that same plan of treatment is being used.

Of course, it will be an oversimplification. That's almost inevitable. But even so, in the next few paragraphs I'm going to set out the main issues in a scheme that you can use as you try to line up the treatment options in your mind, and discuss them with your medical team.

The Risk Benefit Analysis–A Quick Checklist

The whole approach to treatment of any cancer is balancing the potential benefits of a treatment approach against the potential risks—both the consequences and/or the side effects of the treatment, and the risks associated with *not* receiving that treatment.

To make it easier to conceptualize this balancing process, we can use the following checklist of important questions, the ones at the center of the whole approach to the treatment of your particular cancer.

Those questions are:

FIRST, WHAT IS THIS PARTICULAR CANCER LIKELY TO DO IN THE FUTURE IN MY CASE? In many respects, this is the most important question of all in trying to get a grip on your particular situation and what treatment options are appropriate.

What you really want to do is get an idea of what your cancer is like in respect to the following three aspects:

a. Might the cancer recur? Is the chance of it coming back high, or low, or intermediate?

b. Might it spread? Might the cancer metastasize to other parts of the body (for example, the bones or the lungs). And if that is a possibility, is the chance of it happening high, or low, or intermediate?

c. Might it pose a risk to my health or my life? Does this particular cancer represent a threat to your health or your life? If it does, is the size of that threat big, or small, or intermediate? And in what time frame might it do damage: short-term, long-term, or intermediate?

SECOND, WHAT ARE THE TREATMENT OPTIONS, AND WHICH ONES MAY MAKE THE FUTURE BETTER FOR ME? The aim here is to get a handle on the different treatment options, answering the question, "What *could* we do?" before the question, "What *will* we do?" The seven-category system, which follows shortly, will help you with this. And in Part Two we will discuss the various types of treatment in greater detail.

THIRD, WHAT ARE THE RISKS, THE CONSEQUENCES, AND/OR THE SIDE EFFECTS OF THOSE TREATMENT OPTIONS? The aim here is to find out how the proposed treatment option is likely to affect the quality of your life, then for how long.

As you get the basic facts from your medical team, and more information from the pharmacy, and the out-patient treatment unit staff, among others, keep in mind these things:

Some treatment side effects vary. Some side effects are definite and universal: if you have a chemo drug called Adriamycin, for example, you will definitely lose your hair, *and* it will definitely grow back. But with many treatments—radiotherapy is a good example—you may have a lot of skin reaction or you may have none at all. You can predict the amount of skin reaction to a certain extent by how easily you burn when you sit in the sun. But even so the effect may vary.

Which means that you have to ask yourself this question: How much would a particular side effect alter my quality of life?

This is a very personal matter. You have to think about what you do in your daily life and what you enjoy. Then you have to assess the way it would affect you, and how much that would matter to you. The best way to do this is to think about the worst-case scenario: if you got the side effect, what's the worst it could do to your quality of life? Then think of that continuing over the estimated length of time (which is of course just that, an estimate). That will give you some idea of the worst risk from the treatment. And that will make it a bit easier to balance the side effect against the potential benefit.

Let's keep all that in mind as we look at the objectives—the planned benefits—of the treatment plan. So here, is the seven-category system.

The Seven Main Types of Treatment Plans

In this section, I'm going to put it all together, to help you build up an assessment of the risks and benefits in *your* case. To do that, you must first understand the objective of the whole exercise, and ask some important questions. (I know, sometimes it seems the questions will never end. In a way that's true. But each question, and every answer, gets you farther along the path of knowledge and control.)

What is the main objective of the treatment?

Is cure a realistic objective?

Is the idea to try to reduce the chance of the cancer recurring or spreading?

Is the objective to try to control the disease itself?

Is the objective to reduce symptoms caused by the disease?

To help you make sense of this, we are going to divide up the main objectives of treatment into seven broad categories, and I'll give one or two examples of cancer situations in which that treatment approach would be used.

Once again, I realize that I'm oversimplifying a wide spectrum of different treatment plans. But even so, it's worth doing. The details of the treatment plan are often so complicated that it is easy to lose sight of the overall goal. So a reminder of the main game-plan is helpful. It's the map of the forest while you are being handed a catalog of the trees.

In practical terms, then, you can think of the major objective of the treatment plan as being in one of these seven categories:

1. The biopsy or initial surgery is all you need.

There are a few cancers in which, if the cancer is limited to a small area, the biopsy or the initial surgery is all that is necessary at present. In these situations, the area of cancer is very small and is completely contained inside the tissue that was removed at surgery, and in the case of *certain* cancers at this particular stage, the chance of its spreading is zero. In other words, the entire risk has been removed.

This is not a common situation, but it does happen.

Most people are relieved and delighted to hear that they do not need any further treatment. But a few might worry that they are getting substandard treatment, or even that they are being "brushed off" and not getting what they need. So it is worth knowing that this is the correct and standard form of treatment in a few well-defined situations. Here are a few examples:

PRE-INVASIVE CANCER OF THE CERVIX (when the cone biopsy has removed all the malignant cells);

EARLY STAGE COLON OR RECTAL CANCER (when the cancer has not penetrated through the dividing layer of the bowel wall, called the *muscularis mucosa*);

EARLY STAGES OF A TESTICULAR CANCER (in selected cases of both seminoma and nonseminoma, if there is no evidence of spread, including normal tumor marker blood tests, then some centers do not give treatment);

VERY SHALLOW MELANOMA OF THE SKIN (when it is very superficial and has not penetrated through many layers of the skin);

ALL OF THE COMMON SKIN CANCERS (I'm adding this to the list just to be complete. As I noted early in this book, the ordinary skin cancers—squamous and basal cell—are not included in the annual cancer statistics. But it is worth noting that hundreds of thousands of cases of these common cancers are treated each year completely by the initial biopsy, or by local treatment such as freezing with liquid nitrogen.)

2. Some tumor is still present and more surgery is required.
The biopsy has shown an area of cancer and, after the staging tests are done, further surgery is recommended in order to remove the primary tumor, and in many situations to remove the nearby lymph nodes to see if the tumor has spread to them or not. This situation is common, and although it is relatively straightforward it's still worth stressing that in many cases the second surgical operation actually serves two distinct functions: *staging* and *treatment.*

The second or definitive operation may be important not only to establish exactly where the cancer has spread to and where it hasn't (*staging*), but also because it may be, partly or wholly, the definitive *treatment.* The importance of these two distinct functions depends not on the skill or persistence of the surgeon, but on the type of cancer involved. In other words, the importance of the *local* situation depends on the *general* way that the particular cancer behaves.

Take breast cancer as an example. If a woman has a breast cancer that is, say, four centimeters in diameter (not small, but not very big), and if the breast itself is not very large, it might be agreed to do a simple mastectomy (removal of all breast tissue), which is definitive *treatment* for the local mass, and at the same time remove the axillary nodes, which is essential for *staging* of the initial cancer, and planning the treatment. The two parts of the same operation actually do different jobs. Removing the breast tissue treats the breast mass (even though local radiotherapy to the scar may be recommended afterwards), whereas removing the lymph nodes will tell the medical team whether systemic treatment (such as chemotherapy) will be required after surgery. Here are some other examples:

ENDOMETRIAL CANCER. Cancer of the uterus (womb) is usually treated by hysterectomy (removal of the uterus), and in the great majority of cases no further treatment is required.

SARCOMAS. There are many different types of sarcomas, and when they occur in, for example, the muscles of the arm or leg, the standard approach is often to have a second operation in which a larger amount of muscle tissue is removed (often called a *compartmentectomy*). Most centers do not routinely recommend adjuvant chemotherapy after the surgery, but research studies are going on.

BREAST CANCER (A FEW CASES). There are a few situations in which the chance of recurrence is regarded as very low if a mastectomy is done. In these few cases, the standard recommendation would be that no further treatment is required.

BOWEL (COLON OR RECTUM) CANCER (SOME CASES). There are situations in which the biopsy (for example, at colonoscopy) shows a small cancer, and at surgery the entire cancer is removed and there has been no spread to the lymph nodes. In these cases, adjuvant chemotherapy would not necessarily be recommended and follow-up would be all that is required.

3. Tumor is still present: radiotherapy and/or chemotherapy is required.
In this third situation there are two main ways to go: (a) radiotherapy with or without chemotherapy; and (b) chemotherapy as the primary form of treatment.

a. Radiotherapy with or without chemotherapy. There are a number of cancers that are best treated with radiotherapy, chemotherapy, or a combination of both of them, because these approaches either give *better* long-term results than does surgery, or give *equivalent* results without the risks of an operation or the loss of organ function. In some cases, the treatment is with radiotherapy, in others it is chemotherapy, and quite often it is a combination of the two (sometimes referred to as *chemo-rads*).

As with so many treatment plans, the details count for a lot. So try to get a clear understanding of your particular cancer and your particular situation: how the tumor is likely to behave, how treatment options are likely to change that, and what the effects of treatment are likely to be. For example, if chemotherapy and radiation therapy are being recommended together, you need to have a clear understanding of how long each goes on for. Sometimes, for instance, certain chemotherapy drugs are used as what are called *radiosensitizers*, which increase the cancer-killing effect of radiation. Make sure you understand clearly the exact schedule of the treatment and any overlap of one with the other.

Here are some examples of cancers in which radiation therapy (with or without chemotherapy as a strategy to enhance the effect of radiation) is commonly employed:

CERTAIN HEAD AND NECK CANCERS, in particular cancer of the nasopharynx, larynx and hypopharynx;

CANCER OF THE ANAL CANAL;

CANCER OF THE CERVIX:

NON-SMALL-CELL LUNG CANCER;

MANY CASES OF cancer of the esophagus, rectum, vulva, vagina, and penis, along with seminoma, Hodgkin's disease, and non-Hodgkin's lymphoma (some localized cases).

b. Chemotherapy is the primary form of treatment. With some cancers, particularly when the cancer begins in or affects many areas of the body at the same time, chemotherapy is the primary form of treatment because it reaches all parts of the body. Some examples of this include: most types of leukemia; many cases of lymphoma, myeloma, testicular cancer; and certain ovarian cancers.

4. No tumor is present, but adjuvant radiotherapy is helpful.
In this situation all visible tumor has been removed by surgery, but there is a chance of local recurrence (of the tumor coming back in the same area). So you need local radiotherapy to decrease the chance of local recurrence. This situation is quite common, and this approach is highly effective in a high proportion of cases of any type of cancer.

The chance of radiotherapy completely controlling cancer growth in the area, and/or preventing any local recurrence of tumor in that area, depends on how sensitive the tumor cells are to radiation, how big an area needs to be treated, what normal structures happen to be in the radiation fields (such as spinal cord or bowel), and how sensitive those nearby normal tissues are to damage by radiotherapy.

So, in those situations where studies have shown that the chance of local recurrence can be reduced by radiotherapy, then radiotherapy is often recommended as adjuvant therapy (therapy after surgery). Here are some examples:

BREAST CANCER (AFTER LUMPECTOMY OR PARTIAL MASTECTOMY). When the surgery has been more limited (for example, a lumpectomy or partial mastectomy), the chance of the cancer recurring in the scar or in nearby areas of the breast can be reduced by giving radiotherapy.

HEAD AND NECK. There are many situations in head and neck cancers (for example, cancer of the floor of the mouth and tongue) where routine treatment includes radiotherapy after surgery.

BRAIN CANCER (GLIOMAS). Radiotherapy after removal of the tumor (even if all the detectable tumor has been removed) is the standard therapy in most cases.

OTHER SITES: For other examples, see Table 5, pages 254–255.

5. No tumor is present but adjuvant drug therapy (chemotherapy hormones, and/or biologics) is helpful.

Where all visible tumor has been removed but there is a chance of recurrence and spread later on, treatment given now that goes to all parts of the body (*adjuvant systemic treatment*, such as chemotherapy, hormone therapy, and/or biologic therapy) has been shown to decrease the chance of the cancer recurring. This is an important topic: more and more people are being offered adjuvant therapy, and it's important to understand what it is.

Basically, adjuvant treatment means giving treatment *now*, after surgery, to decrease the chance of the cancer recurring *later*. Adjuvant treatment often involves chemotherapy and may make some people feel tired or nauseated or generally under the weather. As one patient on adjuvant therapy observed, "You're making me feel sick now, while I'm well, to increase my chances of staying well and not being sick later." He was right. He had many rough weeks while on this particular adjuvant therapy, but he is perfectly well to this day. He still thinks his description of adjuvant treatment is pretty accurate! Here are a few examples of where adjuvant treatment might be helpful:

BREAST CANCER. The very first research studies that showed the benefit of adjuvant therapy were those done in breast cancer. Depending on whether or not the lymph nodes are involved, whether or not tests on the cancer show that it will likely respond to hormone therapy, (to a certain extent) how aggressive it appears under the microscope, and whether or not it has the molecular target called *her2/neu* on it, adjuvant therapy will be recommended with chemotherapy (of various types), hormone therapy (for example, tamoxifen or an aromatase inhibitor), or biological therapy (with trastuzumab [Herceptin] that binds to the *her2/neu* molecular target on the cancer cell).

BOWEL CANCER (SOME CASES). There is now evidence that if the cancer of the colon or rectum has invaded through most of the bowel wall, or if it has reached a few of the lymph nodes nearby, then giving adjuvant chemotherapy (with drug combinations that often include 5-fluorouracil) will reduce the chance of the cancer recurring.

TESTICULAR CANCER. For teratoma, adjuvant therapy is always recommended if the blood tests (tumor markers) are still abnormal after surgery, and in some circumstances even if they are not.

OVARIAN CANCER EVEN IF ALL DETECTABLE TUMOR HAS BEEN REMOVED AT SURGERY.

SOME OTHER EXAMPLES are included in Table 5, pages 254–255.

6. Watchful waiting.

Sometimes there is no immediate danger. Previously in this book we acknowledged the widespread feeling that, "If it's cancer, it must be treated right away." In fact, there are several cancers where it is now known, as a result of many research studies, that immediate treatment does not make the situation any better, and in these situations studies have shown that the policy of *watchful waiting* is safe and effective. Given the sense of urgency and of emergency that the word *cancer* usually triggers, however, the whole idea of waiting and not treating the cancer immediately can be tough, and can cause some people a great deal of distress and unease.

Here are some examples where watchful waiting is safe and effective:

LOW GRADE (INDOLENT) LYMPHOMA. There are some types of lymphoma (cancer of the lymphatic system) that fluctuate in their growth and progress. They may not change in any way for a very long time—often for several years. So, for example, you might have a lymph node in the neck or the armpit that stays the same size and doesn't alter.

CHRONIC LYMPHOCYTIC LEUKEMIA. The same is also true of chronic lymphocytic leukemia, a slow growing type of leukemia in which many people have no symptoms for years and the only abnormality is a blood count that shows a high number of lymphocytes.

CANCER OF THE PROSTATE. The most common cancer in this category of watchful waiting is cancer of the prostate. The problem, ironically, with cancer of the prostate is that in a very large number of cases, it isn't going to do any major damage in the future. The challenge has been to predict *which* men with cancer of the prostate are *not* going to have trouble. If we could identify them infallibly, then we could spare them the inconvenience of treatment. Although we are not quite there yet, we are making progress. By combining several factors—for example, how aggressive the cancer is (the Gleeson score); how many areas of the prostate are involved; the speed at which the PSA increases; the age of the patient; among other features—it is possible to identify with some confidence those men in whom watchful waiting is safe.

For some other examples, see Table 5, pages 254–255.

7. Treatment for symptom control.
In this situation, I will discuss two areas: (a) where there is still tumor at the site, and you need treatment for that to control or prevent symptons, and (b) there is distant spread and you need treatment to control those symptoms.

a. There is still tumor at the site, and you need treatment for that to control or prevent symptoms. In some situations, it is simply not possible to remove all of the tumor. When that happens, people tend to feel very discouraged and disappointed, but it is very important to listen to what your medical team is telling you. In some of these situations, the cancer is still curable in the long term. And in many others, control may be possible for periods of time.

In this situation, a lot depends on the biology of the particular cancer—in other words, how it is likely to behave and respond to treatment. Since that makes such a considerable difference to the way in which you assess everything (including the risk of severe side effects etc.) I shall divide this subject into two parts:

First, where cure or long-term control is not likely, but medium- or short-term control is very likely.

Second, where long-term control is unlikely, and medium- or short-term control is possible but not very likely.

I have to stress that things change very rapidly in this area, and new treatments are being tested constantly, so this is a topic to discuss with your medical team.

First, where cure or long-term control is not likely, but medium- or short-term control is very likely.

This is a situation that occurs quite frequently. The cancer cannot be removed totally, but is of a type that is quite sensitive to therapy, meaning that the chance of achieving remission is fairly high. When a type of cancer is known to be sensitive to chemotherapy (in other words, if the proportion of cases in which the cancer shrinks or disappears is high), then balancing the potential benefits against potential risks is relatively simpler. Here are a few examples:

SMALL-CELL CANCER OF THE LUNG (SCCL). This has a very high tendency to spread to distant parts of the body, and responds to chemotherapy in the majority of cases. So in most cases of SCCL, the initial surgery may be limited even to a biopsy, and chemotherapy will be recommended soon after. Studies have shown that this is the most effective approach in terms of risk-benefit analysis. More extensive surgery at the outset is not helpful, because the tumor has either spread to other areas already or is likely to do so. And chemotherapy is helpful because it treats all areas, including areas where metastases might be present but are not yet detectable, and has a high chance of success.

CANCER OF THE OVARY (MOST CASES). The situation with cancer of the ovary is similar. Because the cancer begins inside the pelvis and has a high tendency to spread around the abdomen, it is almost always first detected after it has spread. At surgery, the surgeon tries to remove all of the visible cancer, as well as to biopsy other areas where it might be undetectable by the naked eye. Depending, largely, on the nature of that particular cancer (and not on the skill of the surgeon), it might be possible to remove it all, or it might not. In either event, the chance of the cancer recurring or spreading, if it hasn't already done so, is high. As with sccl, the response rate to chemotherapy is also high, which means that it is usually recommended that the patient have several courses of chemotherapy (six, on average) after the surgery, even if there is no disease that is detectable after the operation.

Second, where long-term control is unlikely, and medium- or short-term control is possible but not very likely.

When the cancer is not known to be particularly sensitive to therapy and where the chance of remission is low, you will need to have a detailed discussion with your medical team about the potential benefits and potential side effects of the recommended therapy so that you can make a considered risk-benefit analysis.

This is, of course, a difficult situation, but you do have time to take a breath and think about what is best for you. And in this type of situation, you will want to think about balancing your quality of life with the potential chance of prolonging it with therapy. It is important here that you think through the various different outcomes that could occur.

For example, the best possible scenario would be if the treatment worked and produced a remission of the cancer lasting several or many months with mild and relatively few side effects. If that occurred, it would undoubtedly be advantageous to you, you would have extra time, and that extra time would be of good quality.

At the other end of the scale, the worst case scenario would be that the treatment had no effect on the cancer but did, unfortunately, produce some severe side effects. If that occured, you will lose some of your existing quality of life. So, try to think through how you would respond in both the best case scenario and the worst case scenario.

A lot depends on how you would feel about the potential side effects. For example, if the most common side effects are exhaustion and nausea, how badly would they affect the way you live your life? For some people, nausea is not particularly upsetting, and they can carry on and do most things even during times of queasiness. For others, nausea occupies their entire attention and makes any everyday activity a real trial.

So try to get a picture from your medical team of what the effects are most likely to be, and how you can balance the chance of getting the side effects against the chance of getting a response.

Of course, there is a large measure of uncertainty in this. Nobody can give you a guarantee that the treatment will work or that you will not be troubled by side effects, but going though this thought process can make you better informed, and hopefully you will feel more comfortable with your decision. And that will certainly help you to cope with things.

This type of situation can occur with several types of cancers at the more advanced stages, including cancer of the pancreas, cancer of the esophagus, and advanced melanoma (and for some other examples, see Table 5, pages 254–255).

b. There are symptoms from sites of distant spread. This is also a difficult situation. The cancer has spread to distant areas of the body, and the metastases (secondaries) are of greater concern than is the primary tumor. There are several issues on which you will need clarification to help you make your decision.

First, where are the metastases, and what trouble are they likely to cause you in the near future?

This is important. In some situations, metastases are in a part of the body where they are likely to cause problems soon (the brain is one particular example). In other situations (in certain bones, for example, or with small secondaries in the liver or lungs) it may not be possible to say at the outset whether the metastases are likely to cause problems in the near future or not. So, sometimes, your medical team may suggest waiting for a short time, say a few weeks or so, and then repeating the scan or X-ray to see if the tumors are growing slowly or not. In that way, it will be easier for you to assess what the immediate future is likely to be like, and therefore to make a more informed decision about balancing the value of treatment now *versus* treatment later.

Second, what are the treatment options for treating the metastases? And is the chance of achieving a remission high or low?

The answer to this question depends to a large extent on the type of cancer. For example, in most situations with breast cancer, the chance of achieving remission or response is fairly high, whereas with melanoma the chance of remission is lower. So you need to have an idea of the chance of some success before you can consider the "price" you have to pay in terms of side effects.

Third, what are the likely or expected side effects from the treatment?

This last factor is all about the impact of the treatment on your quality of life. In other words, you will need to have some idea of not just the side effects themselves, but also of the way in which those particular effects would affect you in your day-to-day living.

Thinking through these three aspects of the treatment plan as separate points will help you to balance them in your own mind, and help you to arrive at a practical risk-benefit analysis.

So if you have, let's say, bone metastases from prostate cancer and the recommendation is a hormone treatment with very few side effects, you might well decide to start treatment in the near future since you are unlikely to lose much quality of life.

On the other hand, *if* the cancer is generally resistant to chemotherapy, and *if* the metastases are small, are not causing you any problems now, and are not likely to cause you problems in the immediate future, and *if* the treatment is likely to cause side effects, you might decide to delay the start of therapy.

Once again, I want to stress that in the large majority of cases, the situation is not an emergency. Of course there are occasional emergencies, but they are rare. (For a list of emergency situations, it is worth looking at Table 10.2 in *What You Really Need to Know About Cancer.*)

In general, then, you have time to take a breath and think through the various options. As one of my patients put it, "The treatment is going to go on for several or many weeks; it seems worth spending a little bit of time thinking about it first."

Combining Several Approaches

One final point: there are many cancer situations in which more than one type of treatment is recommended at the same time (or in sequence).

As you will have seen from Step Three, the reason for that is simple: the treatments do different things. For example, a particular cancer might need both local treatment (to decrease the chance of the cancer coming back near the original operation site) and also systemic treatment (treatment that reaches all parts of the body) to decrease the chance of distant spread.

A common example is breast cancer. Suppose a woman is diagnosed with a small cancer of the breast which has spread to a small number of the lymph nodes in the axilla.

If she opts for the more limited surgery (lumpectomy instead of mastectomy) then the standard approach would be to give radiotherapy afterwards because that has been shown to decrease the chance of local recurrence.

However, in addition to that, because the cancer has spread to the lymph nodes, the chance of it later spreading to distant areas of the body is high enough that it is worthwhile using adjuvant systemic therapy (chemotherapy and/or hormone therapy, depending on the characteristics of that particular tumor) as well.

Neither the radiotherapy nor the chemotherapy are better or superior or stronger or more effective. The radiation helps the *local* situation (in the breast and the axilla) and the chemotherapy, or hormone therapy, helps decrease the chance of spread to *distant areas* of the body.

STEP FIVE
"Why Do I Have to Have Follow-up Visits?"
Understanding Prognosis and Monitoring

STEP
FIVE

Everybody finds follow-up visits nerve-racking. And with most cancers, for most of the time, the reasons are easy to understand: you are worried that the cancer might *recur*, and if it doesn't recur you want to know when you can stop worrying and say that you are *cured*.

This section will help you to understand why your follow-up visits are so important and also to cope with the uncertainty and anxiety that surrounds them. It will also help you to understand what is meant by the word *cure*. (In Step Six, which follows, I deal with the issues surrounding the word *recurrence*.)

"When Can I Say I'm Cured?"
Although there is a widely held opinion that you can say you are cured after five years, it is usually not quite as simple or cut-and-dried as that.

The most usual and commonly used definition of the word *cure* is that the disease will "never come back, ever." Using that definition, if there is no evidence of cancer after five years, we can call that a true cure only in a certain number of cancers—those cancers in which we know from long-term studies that if a recurrence has not occurred within five years, it will not occur at all.

In these cancers then—such as cancer of the cervix, cancer of the endometrium, and testicular cancer—if there is no evidence of any recurrence five years after the diagnosis, the cancer will not recur. In the everyday usage of the word, you are *cured*.

For most of the other cancers, however, the chance of recurrence falls steadily, but does not suddenly drop to zero after a certain number of years. It goes down progressively with the passing years. Furthermore, the speed with which the chance of recurrence falls—*and* the point at which one can say "the chance of recurrence is now close to zero"—depends on the type of cancer.

In other words, the point at which one can say, "I am virtually cured" (the chance of that cancer coming back is very close to zero), depends on the type of cancer, and it isn't always five years.

So whereas the situation is simple for cervix, endometrial, and testicular cancers, it is a bit more complex for most of the others.

For example, if you have had breast cancer it is *not* possible to say five years after diagnosis that you are cured. However it *is* possible to say that by ten years after diagnosis, if there is no evidence of recurrence or spread, then the chance of it ever coming back gets very small (close to zero).

In fact one paper reported that in a long-term follow-up study the longest time at which a recurrence occurred was nineteen years after the diagnosis. Now this is not a magical figure; recurrences in the few years *before* that nineteen-year mark were very rare. So for all practical intents and purposes, one could say that ten years after diagnosis the chance of recurrence was very small, at fifteen years after diagnosis it was very, very small and after nineteen years it was zero.

If you had bowel cancer and it had spread to a small number of lymph nodes, if it has not recurred within five years, the chance of it recurring after that is small, and by about seven years or so it is very, very small, and by about ten years or so it is very close to zero.

With small-cell lung cancer, recurrences have a tendency to occur in the first five years but can still occur later. So you could say that at five years the chance of recurrence is low, but, as with many smoking related cancers, the chance of developing a new (a second) cancer of the lung still exists.

I realize that this sounds more complicated than the widely held opinion, "if you're OK at five years, you're cured." But it is such an important factor to take into account with your own particular cancer and your particular situation, that I think it is worth thinking about and discussing (over the course of your many follow-up visits) with your medical team.

Some Other Definitions

Now that I have defined the word *cure*, let me explain what some other commonly used phrases mean.

Complete remission simply means that right now there is no evidence of any cancer when your doctor examines you and does the scans or other tests that originally showed the cancer.

In other words, it means that at this moment all the evidence of cancer has gone. It does not necessarily mean that the cancer will never come back, because as I have just explained, that depends on the type of the cancer.

Partial remission means that the cancer has shrunk. By convention we define a partial remission as when the measurements of the cancer have shrunk to one half, or 50 percent, of what they were.

When we measure cancers on X-rays and scans, we add up two diameters (for example, a vertical and a horizontal) of the measurable tumor and if the *sum* of those two measurements has fallen to 50 percent or less of the original measurements we call it a partial remission.

In many situations, the cancer might remain at exactly the same size. By convention we call any situation in which the tumors remain the same size for six months *prolonged stable disease*.

So those are the definitions of common terms that you will hear during follow-up. And while we are thinking about things you will hear during follow-up, I would like to clear up one other point that very commonly causes misunderstanding (and sometimes dismay).

What a 60 percent Response Rate Actually Means: A Quick Point About Statistics

We all know that statistics are very confusing at the best of times!

When you have a potentially serious illness on the horizon, the high levels of anxiety make it even more difficult to grasp what is actually meant by statements we hear all the time, such as "a 60 percent response rate" or "a 60 percent chance of achieving a partial remission."

A lot of people think that these phrases mean that every patient will experience a 60 percent decrease in the tumor.

But it does not mean that. It means that for every hundred patients treated, sixty will experience a remission. In sixty patients the cancer will shrink to some extent, and in the other forty, unfortunately, the cancer will not be affected by the treatment.

This is an important point. It means that some people (forty out of every hundred in this example) will undergo the treatment and will experience some of the side effects associated with it, but the treatment will have no effect on the cancer.

I am stressing this point not to be negative or pessimistic, but only so that you do not feel that you have been deceived or tricked.

"Why Can't I Have a Test To Tell Me if There's Going To Be a Problem?"

The cancers are actually like most medical conditions, in that the future for any particular person is always a bit uncertain and is not predictable with 100 percent accuracy.

That's the way it is with most diseases. For example, if you had high blood pressure and if you took your medication for it, your blood pressure might now be normal, and your risk of having a stroke might be very close to the risk of the average person. That does not mean you will *definitely not* suffer a stroke. It just means the chance of that happening is only slightly higher than that of the average person.

We are used to understanding and accepting that kind of risk assessment and uncertainty in most medical conditions, but in the case of the cancers we all tend to feel more anxious about the same kind of uncertainty.

Furthermore—and this is a source of considerable disappointment to everyone—there aren't any blood tests or X-rays or scans (at the moment, anyway) that will predict with certainty that the cancer will never come back or spread.

The medical world is working on it and there has been extensive research in this area. But in the great majority of cancers, there is no way of predicting for certain, at an early stage after treatment, that there will not be any problem in the future.

There are routine tests that are done regularly in some but not all cancers (see Table 3, page 242), but many people find it difficult to understand that those tests can only tell you that there is nothing sinister going on *at the moment*. Normal test results (unfortunately called "negative results") are able to tell you that all is well at present. But they cannot predict the future.

The future really depends on the type of cancer, the stage it was at, and other factors such as certain characteristics of the initial tumor, the response to treatment, and so on.

Naturally, everyone resents that feeling of uncertainty, but in the cancers, as in most common diseases, some degree of uncertainty exists. Unfortunately we have to accept that and cope with it, however strongly we dislike it.

Now let us move to discuss the emotions that everybody feels at follow-up visits, together with a strategy that will help you cope.

Worrying About the Follow-up Visits

It is very common for you to feel tense and anxious for the day, even several days, before a follow-up visit. Some people even lose sleep the night before.

The reasons are easy to understand. The clinic becomes associated in your mind with the trauma of diagnosis and of treatment, and even organizing the trip for a follow-up visit can reawaken those feelings.

In fact, it used to be quite common for people who had very bad nausea and vomiting with their chemotherapy to start feeling nauseated on the way to their follow-up visit, even long after the chemotherapy was finished. (Fortunately, the new generations of antinauseant drugs are so good, that this anticipatory nausea is now much rarer and much less severe.)

In some respects the anxiety that many people feel before (and during) each follow-up visit can be compared to fear of flying. It is an emotion (or set of emotions) specifically linked to an event. And the fact that the event, the follow-up visit or the flight, is planned in advance and that there are likely to be many repetitions of it makes the anticipation even worse.

Of course, in the background lurks the fear of hearing bad news, particularly that the cancer has recurred somewhere in your body.

Furthermore, many people feel that any recurrence—wherever and however the cancer comes back—spells the inevitable and rapid end of everything. Actually this fear is so important and such a common source of worry and anxiety, that I've devoted the whole of the next section to that subject.

But here is a novel four-step approach that may help you deal with a rising sense of anxiety at the time of your follow-up visits.

The R.A.C.E. Strategy for Reducing Anxiety

There are a few guidelines that may help you cope with the build-up to any scheduled, tense event. In fact, they are virtually the Golden Rules for dealing with something you dread.

It's called the R.A.C.E. strategy. As one of my patients said, "It *is* a bit like preparing for a race, except it's one that you didn't want to enter, you are nervous about taking part in, and you aren't even sure how you know when you've won."

Recognize the Feeling(s). Recognize the emotions that you are experiencing. Is it pure nervousness? Do you feel jittery? Do you get short-tempered when you're worried? Do you tend to lose your ability to make decisions properly? Do you get angry if you have to drive when you're nervous?

Acknowledge the Emotion(s) to Yourself. Having identified and named the emotion(s) that you're experiencing, it's important to acknowledge them to yourself. It's often worth actually saying it out loud (which is better if you're alone, though nowadays if anyone does see you they'll assume you're on a cell phone!). Say to yourself, "I'm feeling nervous because I'm going to the clinic tomorrow," or "I was really annoyed about that little thing because I'm worried about the visit this afternoon."

Calming Strategies. Take one or two practical steps that make you feel calmer. Maybe take a friend with you, take a tranquilizer before you go, have someone else drive you there, write down the important questions you wish to ask, and leave some room for the answers.

Enjoy Something Afterwards. Give yourself a special treat after the visit. Go to a movie, have lunch with a friend and go shopping together. It's probably better to do that after the visit, because if you do it before, you might be preoccupied with the visit and not enjoy the treat.

The whole point about the R.A.C.E. strategy is that it gives you something to do—an approach that you can use to fill the nervous void. And it changes the experiences associated with the visit. After a few times, just as with fear of flying, the strategy reduces the sense of dread and foreboding until a follow-up visit becomes almost routine.

It takes time, but it happens!

STEP SIX
"What If It Recurs…?"

Although this book is intended to help you through the first few weeks after a cancer diagnosis, it might help you even in that early period to have a framework of thoughts and plans for the possibility of recurrence, even though that is quite unlikely to happen in the first few weeks. So I make no apologies for dealing with recurrence here. We can talk about how we would handle an elephant in the room—a looming presence that everyone knows is there but no one actually talks about—even though there's no elephant there now, and there may never be. Making plans for an eventuality, however unlikely, actually helps a great deal.

Recurrence is a thought—or fear—that almost everybody thinks about every time they come to the clinic, and in between visits, too. It's a genuine elephant in the room.

"Is Recurrence 'Game Over'?"

The possibility of the cancer returning causes enormous of anxiety. This is not inappropriate. It *is* a worry, particularly since there is a widespread impression that any type of recurrence of any type of cancer will inevitably and immediately cause immediate deterioration or even death. Almost especially because everybody has a general feeling that if the cancer ever comes back, it's bound to be game over.

Actually it isn't.

As I've said, and repeated, and reinforced, throughout this book, the cancers are a group of diseases, each of which has a characteristic pattern of behavior that is different from the others. And this also applies to recurrence. In some cancers, recurrence can be very significant, in many others it is much less so and the situation may still be curable.

In fact, the significance of a recurrence depends on two main factors: the type of the cancer and the type of recurrence—whether it is a *local* recurrence at the site of the original tumor or nearby, or *distant* recurrence (a metastasis); for example, in an organ or area some distance from the tumor.

These two aspects largely determine the type of treatment that is recommended, the chance of that treatment being effective against the cancer, and whether or not a cure or long-term control is still possible.

There is a wide range of situations related to tumor recurrence. And as always with any of the cancers, it will help if you can get a more accurate and practical handle on the situation in your own particular case. That may help reduce that sense of dread.

When Should You Find Out What the Next Options Are?

A question that might occur to you as you think about this topic is "How should I prepare myself for something that might not happen?" And actually how you handle and cope with a hypothetical eventuality is very much a personal matter: it has to do with the way you cope generally with things that threaten you, and what strategies you use to minimize the anxiety and worry caused by those threats.

In other words, how you cope with this type of worry relates to your own personal coping strategies—the things you usually do and have done in your past.

Some people like to find out what could be done in every worst-case scenario, some people simply like to know that there are options which can be discussed if the need arises.

If you happen to be the kind of person who can't sleep easy without knowing more, then I think it's reasonable to ask your medical team during the follow-up period what would happen if the tumor recurred and what treatment options there are.

I would recommend—and this is a personal opinion, there is no right or wrong—that you discuss this after the initial course of treatment. At an early stage in the treatment, both you and your medical team are likely to have a lot of things to cope with anyway. When you are in the follow-up phase—which, don't forget, can be thirty years or more—you will probably find that you can cope with the discussion more easily.

"What's Treatment Like?"

How Cancer Is Treated

In this Part, I will give you a broad overview of the main types of treatment and how they are likely to affect you.

In particular, I will explain how the treatment is used, what the most common side effects are, and how you will feel. In other words, how any particular treatment is likely to affect the way you live your life.

Of course, the range is very wide: some cancers are treated by taking a tablet every day, and there are few side effects. Other cancers require surgery, followed by chemotherapy and radiotherapy—each of which will have some effect on you. In rare situations, there are some cancers, such as some leukemias and myeloma, which are best treated with high dose treatments and, for example, bone marrow transplants. These may require several weeks in hospital over a period of time, with a recovery period of a few months. So the range is very wide, and you shouldn't be put off or scared by what you read in this section if it doesn't apply to you.

But if you get at least the general concepts from what you read here, you will be better prepared to understand the specific details of your particular treatment.

I will describe each of the four main types of treatment for the cancers—surgery, radiotherapy, chemotherapy, and biological therapy. For each one I will explain generally what is involved, mentioning some of the most common side effects so you can be aware of them. But remember that side effects will vary with the specific treatments that are recommended in your own case.

This part of the book is therefore going to be experiential: what it feels like, how it may alter your life, and what you can expect.

Surgery

Surgery is the oldest known form of treatment for cancer. There are descriptions of mastectomy for breast cancer in Egyptian hieroglyphic writings, so the history of cancer surgery is more than five thousand years old.

"How Does Surgery Work?"
The idea behind surgery is easy to understand: the objective is to remove a particular cancer, or as much of it as possible, while doing as little as possible to disturb the neighboring normal tissues and organs of the body.

"What Is Surgery Like?"
Of course, the range of surgical operations is very wide, so there isn't a single or simple answer to the question, "What is surgery like?"

In most areas of the body, a tumor can be removed partly or totally. What the operation is like depends predominantly on three things:

First, which part of the body is involved, and therefore what normal organs or tissues are nearby. Second, how the cancer is attached to neighboring tissues and how wide the operation needs to be to remove it. Third, in what way, and how completely, normal structure and function can be reconstructed or re-established after the tumor is removed.

So as your surgical team describes and discusses the operation with you, make sure that you understand: where the tumor is (as far as the scans and other tests can define it), which nearby organs are likely to be disturbed during surgery, and what restoration of structure and function can be done.

How quickly you recover from any surgery depends not only on the type of operation, but also on your own medical condition, and on other medical factors such as your age, general state of health, and any other medical conditions you may have.

Your surgeon can thus only *estimate* how quickly you will recover. And you may be given a range rather than an exact number of days. Let me illustrate the range with a couple of examples.

At the lesser end of the scale, there is the operation to remove a breast lump.

This operation is called a *lumpectomy*, or sometimes a *partial mastectomy* and is most often accompanied by another small operation on the armpit in which some of the lymph nodes are removed so that they can be examined to see if the cancer has spread there. This part is called *axillary dissection* or *axillary node sampling* or *sentinel node biopsy*, depending on the objective and the extent of the operation.

The complete procedure—lumpectomy plus axillary node sampling—is generally regarded as a fairly small operation because there are no major organs or systems in the area. Hence recovery—in the sense of "getting back on your feet"—can be fairly short, sometimes two or three days. Some patients want to go home within a day. This operation is representative of the minor types of surgery.

At the other end of the scale, however, there are major operations on the abdomen or major operations on the chest, after which you should plan for a longer recovery period—usually several weeks. As the incision heals over the first few days, activities such as moving around and coughing steadily become less painful and less uncomfortable, and you will find that you can gradually do more. So the time to get back on your feet after major surgery is usually three or more weeks. The time needed to get back to normal may be two or three times that long. How soon you can return to work depends on your general state of health, what physical activities are involved in your work, and perhaps on such factors as whether or not your employer can accommodate part-time work, for example.

Here is a list of the approximate time it takes to get back on your feet. The time to begin feeling nearly normal or resuming work is almost always much longer.

BREAST SURGERY	3–7	DAYS
LUNG SURGERY	2–4	WEEKS
MINOR ABDOMINAL SURGERY	1–3	WEEKS
MAJOR ABDOMINAL SURGERY	2–4	WEEKS
PELVIC SURGERY	2–4	WEEKS
CRANIOTOMY	1–2	WEEKS

These times are approximate only. Nevertheless, the more you know about the planned surgery, the better prepared you will be. And the more you understand about the nature and the purpose of the operation, the better able you'll be to cope after it.

Surgical Operations for Staging the Cancer

With many cancers, it is important to know exactly how far the cancer has spread locally and whether it has, for example, spread to the local lymph nodes. In many cases, but not all, the treatment for larger or widespread cancers is different from that of more localized or smaller cancers.

So in some cases, often after CT scans or MRI scans, it may be recommended that further staging be done by an operation, so that treatment can be more accurately planned. This is not undertaken lightly. Your surgical team should be able to explain very clearly the reasons for your needing to have any staging operation.

(In Table 4, page 253, I've shown the most common types of cancer in which staging surgery is often used.)

"What Side Effects Can I Expect?"

The after effects of surgery depend on many of the same factors we have just described: which part of the body is being operated on; how extensive the operation needs to be (which depends partly on how far the cancer has spread and whether or not it is impinging on neighboring organs); and how much reconstruction can be done afterwards.

Try to get from your surgical team a general impression of what your life will be like after the first two or three weeks, when the tissues have mostly healed.

Now almost everybody wants to be above average and to recover faster than everyone else. But I suggest that you not set the bar too high. Having unrealistic expectations of your recovery or aiming at targets that you can't reach will lead to disappointment. Set a steady pace for your recovery and be rewarded with gradual progress.

"What About Long-Term Effects?"

After surgery, as the saying goes, "some parts are gone, and some are in a different place." The long term effects of any particular operation depend on which organ systems have been affected and what reconstruction has been done or will be done.

Here are a few types of surgery with their most common consequences:

AFTER BOWEL (COLON) SURGERY. The effects depend on how much of the colon has been removed, but it is quite common to experience a change in your bowel habit. The stool tends to be softer and sometimes fluid, and many people find that after surgery their bowel habit is affected more easily by what they eat (variations in their diet) than it was before the surgery.

AFTER STOMACH OR PANCREATIC OR BILE DUCT SURGERY. Surgery in any of these areas may affect the way your gastrointestinal system copes with and digests the food you eat. It often happens that food seems to go "straight through" and you may feel the urge to defecate soon after eating. If the bile duct system is affected, you may have difficulty digesting fat, and the stools may become pale and bulky and may smell unusual. If the pancreas is affected, you may also have difficulty digesting several types of food—this is called *malabsorption*—and you may have to take pills containing pancreatic enzymes with your food.

AFTER PROSTATE SURGERY. Depending on the type of operation, there is the possibility of erectile dysfunction in the long term. Urinary incontinence is usual in the short term and usually resolves or improves greatly after several weeks. Sometimes the urinary incontinence only happens during a stress, such as coughing or straining while lifting heavy objects.

AFTER HEAD AND NECK SURGERY. Depending on which part of the mouth, throat or neck has been operated on, you may experience changes in the voice, or in swallowing. If it seems likely that your voice will be affected, you may be referred to a speech therapist, even before the operation.

AFTER BREAST SURGERY. Most patients who have had axillary node sampling will afterwards have some degree of frozen shoulder. You will be given some exercises aimed at restoring the full mobility of the affected shoulder, and it's worth taking them seriously and doing them as recommended.

"What Does It Mean When The Doctor Says 'We Got It All'?"

In the whole area of cancer treatment the reason why additional treatment may be required after surgery is possibly the most common cause of misunderstanding.

The general public is becoming remarkably well informed about the cancers and nowadays more and more people realize that treatment may be required after surgery. But it is still an important area of discussion.

In that discussion, one simple fact is critical: whether or not further treatment is required after surgery depends on the type of the cancer and the stage it is at, not necessarily on the skill of the surgeon!

If, for example, a cancer of the bowel (colon) has spread to the local lymph nodes that lie alongside neighboring parts of the bowel, that is a signal that this particular cancer has a tendency to spread later on to other parts of the body, particularly the liver. Over the last two decades, many clinical studies have shown that if you give treatment after the operation as insurance—adjuvant therapy—the chance of the cancer spreading is considerably reduced.

This has nothing to do with the operation or with the surgeon. All the lymph nodes have (usually) been removed, but the fact that the cancer had spread to them indicates that this particular cancer has a high tendency to spread. And clinical studies have shown that adjuvant therapy reduces the chance of new tumors later on.

So if the surgeon told you, "We got it all," he or she is quite correct in that all visible tumor has been removed. Even so, there is a chance that the cancer will recur and spread (from cancer cells that are not detectable by any means known to us at the moment) and *for that reason*, and nothing to do with the nature of the surgery, more treatment is recommended.

Other types of therapy, such as radiation therapy and chemotherapy, may also be used after surgery. There are several cancers—for example, cancers of the breast, the colon, and the ovary—where it has been shown that, first, even after excellent surgery, in which all the visible parts of the tumor have been removed, there is still a fair chance that the cancer will recur, and second, that giving treatment after the surgery can reduce this chance. I need to emphasize once again (and very clearly) that this does not imply that the surgery was unnecessary or was substandard in any way. It means that after normal (even exemplary) surgery, there is still a chance of the cancer coming back, and research studies have shown that this chance can be reduced by giving adjuvant therapy. Adjuvant therapy is dictated by the particular type of cancer and its response to therapy after surgery, and the need for it does not imply anything about the surgery, or the surgeon.

When Surgery Is Not an Option: "Why Can't They Try an Operation Anyway?"

Most people feel, sometimes appropriately, that surgery is the mainstay and first option for all cancers—that if the problem is *cancer*, there should be a type of surgery that could *remove* it.

Depending on the type of the cancer and where it is, however, surgery is not always feasible. We can usefully think of these circumstances under two headings: recurrence or spread of the primary tumor, and those situations in which the tumor mass cannot safely be removed.

As regards recurrence of the primary tumor there are some cases in which surgical removal does actually help. If a breast cancer recurs in the scar or in neighboring areas of the breast, for example, it may still be possible to achieve long-term control by removing the recurrence. There are similar situations in some colon and rectal cancers, and a few situations in cancer of the cervix.

For most of the other cancers, unfortunately, this is not true: surgery does not help the long term outlook.

Nor is surgery usually helpful in most sites of secondary spread. Surgery is generally not feasible, except under exceptional and unusual circumstances, for secondary cancers in the lungs, or in the liver, or for multiple recurrent cancers of the ovary.

So the biology of the cancer and the part of the body affected sometimes means that surgery is not feasible, and this is almost always difficult for patients and relatives to understand and accept.

However, these are the very situations in which further treatment options need to be discussed and considered carefully. Some of these cancers may still be responsive to, for example, chemotherapy or hormone therapy, and it is possible to achieve control of the disease for a period of time, sometimes for relatively prolonged periods. In these situations, it is important that you get a clear understanding of any possible benefit from any treatment, and of the likelihood and nature of the possible side effects.

There is a second situation where surgery is not possible: when the entire tumor cannot be removed without serous hazard, and only a partial removal would therefore be possible.

There are several circumstances where such an operation would involve cutting through the tumor itself. Although this may sound better than nothing, in fact it is almost always extremely hazardous. Because cancer cells don't make scar tissue, any such operation would produce an operation site that would never heal or one where abnormal channels (fistulae) might form between, for example, the bowel and other pelvic organs. So in many of these situations (a tumor in the pelvis, for example) if the tumor cannot be removed in its entirety, then a partial removal with a cut-through is actually very hazardous and would not even allow the operation site to heal satisfactorily.

Hence, sometimes surgery is not feasible, and although this is initially very disappointing, it does avoid severe complications and symptoms. Having said that, however, I must add that there are a few circumstances where a partial removal of a tumor is safe—in brain tumors, for example. It may happen that part of a brain tumor is too close to very important normal structures and so the tumor cannot be removed in its entirety. In those and similar (although rare) circumstances, removing as much of the tumor as possible is the standard practice.

Common Myth: "If The Air Gets to the Cancer, It Will Spread"
This is a very old myth indeed. In fact in the late Victorian era, it was widely believed that operating on a cancer accelerated its spread and hastened the patient's death.

This happens to be complete nonsense.

The idea made intuitive sense way back then, because most cancers were not diagnosed until they were very big. The Victorians did not have X-rays and CT scans, or even regular health checkups, so people would persevere with their daily life as symptoms or lumps began and progressed. Only when daily life, particularly work, was impossible did they seek medical help.

Furthermore, surgical operations in those days were fearsome—in terms of pain, postoperative complications, and expense. So even when an operation was recommended, people postponed it. At the time of surgery it was quite possible that the patient's total tumor burden might have been several kilograms (see the diagram in *What You Really Need to Know About Cancer*)—only a few weeks or months from the end of the patient's life—a situation that was made much worse by the very high rate of complications, infection, and mortality in the postoperative period.

By the time cancer masses total one or two kilograms, they have usually progressed more than seven eighths of their total course.

So you can see that, early on, surgery was associated in the public's mind with imminent death.

Even today, in those rare situations where a cancer grows very rapidly, people sometimes talk about surgery as if it were somehow the cause, and not simply the means by which the diagnosis was made.

Nowadays, that particular myth is fading away. But it still has a few echoes and small ripples, and can occasionally cause distress and doubt to patients and friends.

Radiation Oncology (Radiotherapy)

Radiation was first discovered by Pierre and Marie Curie in the 1890s and within a few years, physicians were holding lumps of radium against cancerous masses in the breast.

"How Does Radiotherapy Work?"

Radiation, or *radiation therapy* as it is called when it is being used in the treatment of the cancers, means using high-energy electromagnetic waves to kill cells. In many ways, the radiation used in cancer treatment is similar to imaging X-rays, but the radiation contains much higher energy and the radiation beams are therefore capable of doing much more damage to the cells exposed to it. Both visible light and ultraviolet rays are also electromagnetic waves, which is why if the skin is damaged during radiation the effects are very similar to sunburn.

Radiation therapy is used to cure some cancers and to treat others. Radiation can also be used to reduce symptoms.

The rays used for radiotherapy are created in two ways. In most circumstances they are created artificially using devices rather like old fashioned television cathode-ray tubes, or (most often nowadays) by radiotherapy machines, including ones called *linear accelerators*. Or they are produced inside devices that contain naturally radioactive substances such as cobalt. The rays created by these two different methods have different characteristics. In particular, depending on which machine they come from, they penetrate through human tissues to different extents and, therefore, do different amounts of damage to the areas around the tumor.

This is an important difference. For example, if the radiation is generated by a low-voltage machine, the rays give up most of their energy very near the surface and do not penetrate very far. These rays can therefore be used very effectively for skin tumors. High-energy radiation, on the other hand, penetrates further and may give the highest dose of radiation deep below the surface. It is thus extremely important for the radiation oncologist to work out exactly where the tumor is, so that the maximum dose of radiation can be delivered close to the tumor, sparing as much as possible of the normal surrounding tissue.

The radiation given off by the machines is measured with great accuracy, and tested and monitored very closely so that the dose of radiation given out by each machine per treatment is known precisely.

The radiation is given to the area of the tumor (the field) and this is where the skill and expertise of your radiation oncologist and the technology in the radiotherapy department come into play.

The dose of radiation depends on two factors. First, the dose should be high enough to produce the maximum cancer-killing effect. That depends on the type of the cancer: some cancers are more sensitive to radiation than others. It depends also on the objective of the therapy: radiation that is given with the objective of curing the cancer, for example, may require a higher dose than radiation which is intended to reduce pain.

The second factor is the normal tissues in the area. Some normal tissues are not easily affected by radiotherapy: bone, for example, is relatively insensitive to radiation, so that higher doses can be given without producing damage. Other tissues, such as the spinal cord, are very sensitive to potential damage, and doses have to be carefully controlled and given in ways that will minimize that damage. In addition to the spinal cord, there are other tissues and organs that require particular care and attention when radiotherapy is being planned— including the lining of the digestive tract (esophagus, small intestine, and colon, for example), the lungs, kidneys, and eyes.

So in planning any radiotherapy treatment, the radiation oncologist considers the type and site of the tumor, and then carefully works out which normal tissues are likely to be exposed to the radiation given to that area.

This is why the process of *planning* radiation therapy is so important.

Understanding Planning: "What's the First Visit Like?"
The key to good results with radiation therapy is giving as much radiation as possible to the cancer cells, while exposing normal tissues and structure to as little radiation as possible. And the key to that is knowing as accurately as possible where the tumors are, through planning, limiting the radiation as far as possible to those areas only.

So the whole process that we call *planning* is all about getting the best possible results in your particular case. There are several steps in the planning process and if you know a bit about them in advance you'll be less baffled and bewildered by the process.

Imaging
At your first visit to a radiation therapy department, you'll be assessed by the radiation oncologist (or a member of her or his team) who'll be overseeing your therapy.

At that first assessment, there will usually be a review of your medical records, and often various points in your history and/or physical examination will be checked.

Depending on your situation, your radiation oncologist may consult with other oncologists, or a pathologist, or other specialists (in a multi-disciplinary consultation).

The radiation team will also look at the X-rays and scans that have already been done. Quite often, additional CT scans (and sometimes MRI scans or other specialized imaging techniques such as arteriograms) may be required. So if additional imaging tests are required, it's because it really matters. The more accurate the assessment of the cancer, the more effective and the safer the radiation will be. Perfecting the planning is the biggest factor in getting good treatment for you, so please be patient, even though it may feel irritating and unnecessary from your point of view.

In some cases, further blood tests may also be required, often to ensure that various organ systems are working properly and to avoid as far as possible any damage to any system that is not perfect.

The Radiation Field

So in planning your therapy, your radiation oncologist starts by working out where the tumor is and how big an area needs to be included in the area of radiation, or the *radiation field*.

Then, the oncologist has to work out what other structures and tissues are likely to be included in the field—for example, bowel, spinal cord, skin, and so on. Then the type of radiation can be selected that will give the maximum dose to the area of the tumor and the minimum to the surrounding normal tissue.

Next, the oncologist works out the best method of giving the radiation—in other words, into how many doses (fractions) it needs to be divided. This depends on several factors—mostly, again, on how wide an area is to be included in the field and on the nearby normal tissues and how sensitive they are. If the area is small and in a relatively insensitive tissue such as bone, the radiation may be given all in one fraction.

But a high dose of radiation aimed at curing a tumor in a breast, by contrast, usually requires many fractions—up to twenty or twenty-five.

Then, there are different ways to spread out radiation exposure over different areas, where the tumor, not the normal tissue, catches the brunt of the radiation each time. This is the idea behind giving the radiation from two or more different directions (radiation beams). The arrangements of the beams are computer generated by a treatment planning team made up of radiation physicists and technologists (called *radiation therapists*) in consultation with the oncologist.

Using carefully positioned beams, the skin to the left and the right of the tumor, for example, gets less than half of the radiation (or much less depending on the penetration of the rays), while the cancer gets the full brunt.

Markings

In order to make sure that the radiation is given to exactly the same place each time, it may be necessary for the technologists to make ink marks on your skin so that the rays can be lined up with perfect accuracy each time. Since all ink marks on skin disappear in a few days as the skin grows and replaces itself, it some cases it may be necessary to make a small indelible tattoo on the skin. In certain areas of the body, it may be necessary to make a plastic mould or mask to hold the tissues in exactly the same place each time. If that is necessary your radiation oncologist will explain the full details.

"What Is The Treatment Like?"

From your point of view, the radiation treatment itself is similar to having an ordinary X-ray—there's very little to it.

Radiation is usually given in small daily doses called *fractions*. For each fraction, you will be shown to a room in which resides the particular radiation machine appropriate for the therapy planned for you.

(By the way, there's a diagram of what a radiation therapy machine and room look like in *What You Really Need to Know About Cancer.*) You can get a very realistic and helpful virtual tour of a radiation department (in fact it's the radiation department at the Princess Margaret Hospital) on the Web site at www.uhn.ca. It is very easy to use and will help prepare and reassure you before your first visit to any radiation department. I strongly recommend that you visit the site.

Your radiation therapist will help you lie down on a flat table and line up the machine over the area, just as if you were having an X-ray taken. (Which is, basically, the same thing, except that the dose of radiation from an X-ray is much lower.) The therapist will then leave you for a few minutes, and the machine will be turned on for the exact length of time necessary—usually a couple of minutes—by the technologist, who will monitor the whole process from the control unit. While the machine is on, you must keep still but you will not feel any effects. There is no pain or heat or smell or noise. (Some people briefly experience the "fresh air" smell of ozone, which is formed in minute quantities during radiation, but most don't.) In other words, it is very similar to having an X-ray taken.

Customarily, the dose fractions are given on each weekday. Each daily dose is called a *fraction*, and the dose of radiation is measured in units called *centi-Grays* or *cGy*. Thus, a typical total dose of radiation might be 5000 cGy. That total dose is split into daily fractions. So you might be told that you will get 50 Gray in 20 fractions, meaning that you will get a total dose of 50 Gray (5000 cGy) in 20 small doses, each of which will be 250 cGy.

Each dose takes a couple of minutes or so. Usually, taking into account the setting up of the machines and so on, you will probably need to allow up to an hour or an hour and a half for each dose, from the time you arrive at the radiation center to the time you leave.

"What Side Effects Can I Expect?"

While the radiation is being given you won't experience anything. The later side effects of the radiation depend on the total dose (the number of centi-Grays) given, the area of the body being treated, and the number of daily doses or fractions used to deliver the complete treatment.

The easiest way to think of the side effects is to divide them into general side effects that may occur in any radiation treatment, and specific side effects related to the particular area of the body being treated.

The *general* side effects that may occur with any radiation treatment include:

SKIN. Later on—usually a few days later—your skin in the area that has been irradiated may tingle and then turn red like sunburn. Sometimes the skin reaction can be quite severe for several days, and occasionally there may be temporary blisters or ulcers. In most cases, however, there is no skin reaction at all.

FATIGUE. A feeling of fatigue or tiredness is quite common, particularly if the radiation fields are large or if the program of treatment takes several weeks.

HAIR LOSS. You will have hair loss *only* in the areas being treated. So chest hair is lost in the radiation field if you're having lung radiation, and armpit hair is lost if you are having the armpit treated as part of your breast cancer treatment. It's important to know that hair loss caused by radiation is permanent only if high doses are received by the hair follicle.

NAUSEA. Generally, nausea is rare unless large areas of your abdomen or you liver are being radiated.

Other side effects depend on which area of your body is getting the radiation, and it is always worthwhile checking with your radiation oncologist about the specific problems that may be associated with radiation in the particular part of your body being treated. Particular organs such as the spinal cord need special attention. Problems develop rarely, but it is helpful for you to know what to look out for.

The local effects of radiotherapy include:

SKIN. In most cases, there will be some effects on the skin that's in the radiation field. Sometimes the effects on the skin are virtually negligible. In most cases, they are similar to mild or moderate sunburn, and in a small number of cases, particularly if you have been sensitive to the sun in the past, they may be like bad sunburn, occasionally with some blistering and oozing. These effects all heal within a few weeks, sometimes leaving behind little freckles or mottled pigment changes, and occasionally tiny red veins in the area.

HAIR. As I mentioned, hair that is part of the radiation field is likely to be lost. It may grow back later, but very often it doesn't. So it is important for you to be aware that the area of treatment—and nowhere else!—is likely to become, and to remain, hairless after the treatment.

DIGESTIVE TRACT. If the radiation field includes the abdomen and/or the liver, you are quite likely to experience some nausea, sometimes with some vomiting. You quite likely will have some diarrhea, which may continue for several days or a couple of weeks. If the field includes the gullet or esophagus, you will likely experience some discomfort or pain on swallowing, again for several days or a few weeks.

MOUTH, RECTUM, VAGINA. All of these areas are lined with mucous membranes and can be quite sensitive to radiation. You may get ulcers in the area, which steadily heal, although they can be very uncomfortable for several days.

"What About Long-Term Effects?"

SKIN. Generally speaking, skin in the radiated area tends to remain a little darker than the neighboring areas and sometimes looks a bit freckled or mottled. If that happens to you, be reassured that it is completely normal! However, when the dose to the skin is very high, the pigment-forming cells can actually die and leave the area quite light, somewhat similar to a mild case of the skin condition known as *vitiligo*.

LYMPHEDEMA. If radiation involves the upper part of the arm or of the leg, some degree of swelling (called *lymphedema*) of the limb can occur. It is actually quite common to have some degree of swelling, with the girth of the affected arm being more than two centimeters larger than the opposite arm, for example. Medically speaking, the swelling is not serious. And it certainly does *not* mean—as many people fear—that the cancer is recurring. But the cosmetic effect and the slight feeling of heaviness can be very annoying. Some centers have lymphedema clinics, and many others have clinical nurse specialists who can advise and recommend various measures to improve the situation.

FIBROSIS. Certain areas of the body—inside the lungs or inside the abdomen, for example—may form scar tissue after several kinds of treatment, including radiation. Hence scarring, called *fibrosis*, can occur after radiotherapy to the lungs, in the abdomen, in the skin, and in several other areas.

The symptoms depend on which areas are affected. In the lung, for example, you may notice shortness or breath or a dry cough or both. In the abdomen you may have intermittent episodes of abdominal pain, sometimes partial obstruction of the bowel. In the skin, fibrosis feels like a scar under the surface of the skin and may change the contour of that part of the area as you see it. It may also affect the movement and mobility of that area, for example, around the shoulder.

INFERTILITY. In both males and females, sterility can occur, meaning that you could become infertile. In a few situations, there are measures that can be used to prevent infertility, or to get around it, such as sperm banking. But this may not always be possible. In some cases, infertility may have been produced by the disease process itself before treatment commenced.

SECOND MALIGNANCIES. Like many forms of therapy that attack the nucleus of the cells, radiation therapy can increase the chance of your later developing another type of cancer. After more than two decades following radiation therapy, the chance of getting a second cancer (for example of the thyroid, or breast, or sarcoma of the skin) is increased very slightly.

In general terms, depending on the area and the type of treatment, your medical team may recommend exercise programs or other forms of therapy to decrease the effects described above. It's really worth taking those recommendations seriously.

Common Myth: Radiation Damages the Immune System and Does More Harm Than Good

This is a myth, one that has no foundation in fact whatsoever. But it is quite persistent and can worry new patients.

Who knows where the myth started! Perhaps it started because radiation is often given to the lymph nodes in the neighboring regions of the body (the armpit for breast cancer), and lymph nodes are part of the immune system. (But, of course, the armpit nodes represent a tiny, almost negligible proportion of the body's immune system.)

For whatever reason, the impression grew that people who had everyday radiation therapy could develop suppression of the immune system and this might make it easier for the cancer to recur or spread.

This is—to put it plainly—nonsense.

In the case of any cancer, studies show that people who have had radiation do *not* have an increased chance of recurrence. Quite the contrary: where radiotherapy is used as part of the routine treatment, the chance of local recurrence of the cancer is greatly reduced. The myth that radiation somehow makes things easier for the cancer is without any foundation in fact.

Chemotherapy

The modern era of chemotherapy actually started during World War II, when a cargo ship carrying mustard gas (used in World War I) exploded. Many who survived the blast died in the weeks following because their bone marrow was destroyed by the gas. Mustine—the first chemotherapy drug produced, after the war—was designed as a variant of mustard gas, and was found to be dramatically effective in hitherto untreatable advanced Hodgkin's disease.

"How Does Chemotherapy Work?"
Chemotherapy drugs kill cells that are actively growing and multiplying.

The drugs that we call *chemotherapy drugs* (sometimes also called *cytotoxic agents*) make up a varied group of chemical agents, but they all have this one thing in common: they kill cells that are actively multiplying and reproducing. Generally, there is a higher proportion of reproducing cells inside a cancer than in normal tissue. Hence, generally, chemotherapy drugs do more damage to cancers than they do to normal tissues. Which is why they are used.

If cells are growing and multiplying, they can be damaged by chemotherapy: that's good if they are cancer cells, but it's a hazard if they are your normal cells in the bone marrow, mouth, hair and other tissues. That is why most chemotherapy drugs have so many side effects. That is why the dosage has to be so carefully controlled, and also why the difference between a dose that is effective against the cancer, and a dose that has major side effects is often very slight.

Chemotherapy Drugs and the Growth of Cells

Over the years, research has shown that there are many different ways in which chemotherapy drugs can interfere with—or stop—cells multiplying. They can interfere with the cells assembling building blocks to make new DNA, assembling the components for the DNA, separating the duplicated chromosomes during division, and so on.

By whichever of these mechanisms the chemotherapy drug works, the objective is always the same: to stop growing cells from duplicating.

This is a very good thing when it applies to cancers. Cancer cells that cannot reproduce cannot grow and spread.

However, there are many organs and systems in your body in which growth and multiplication is important, and hence, the side effects of many chemotherapy drugs. For example, the cells in your bone marrow are constantly growing and producing the various components of your blood—the red cells, the white cells, and the platelets. The cells lining your gastrointestinal tract and your mouth are also constantly growing and producing new cells to maintain the lining of the gut. Your hair grows constantly because the cells in the hair follicles are reproducing and manufacturing new hair. In the testicles, the sperm progenitors are also multiplying to produce new sperm. All of these normal cell activities—and some others besides—can be affected to a greater or lesser extent by chemotherapy agents.

In this way, chemotherapy agents are very different from most other medications. For example, antibiotics are used to kill bacteria, and bacterial cells are basically like plant cells and have a very different structure from our body cells. So antibiotics do not generally interfere with the functioning of our normal cells.

But cancer cells, unlike bacterial cells, are very similar to normal cells. So that drugs that damage cancer cells are highly likely to damage the normal cells also.

All of this means that, even with the most sensitive cancers and the best drugs, the margin for error is small.

Most chemotherapy drugs may kill the patient if they are given in relatively slight excess—at, say, twice the normal dose. By contrast, in treating bacterial infections with common antibiotics, there would usually be no lethal or serious side effects at even ten times the normal dose.

For all these reasons, then, chemotherapy drugs—more than almost any other groups of drugs in the medical armory—need to be monitored closely and must be given only by experienced oncologists.

"What Is Chemotherapy Like?"

Chemotherapy drugs are most commonly either given in tablet form by mouth, or injected into a vein. The injection can be a single shot (the medical term is *bolus*) lasting a few minutes, or an infusion, which drips in larger volumes of fluid over several hours.

The drugs can also be injected into the abdominal cavity (peritoneum), into the cerebro-spinal fluid (csf), into an artery (rarely), subcutaneously under the skin, or (very occasionally) may be applied as a cream to the skin.

(Some drugs can be given in more than one way, so I've set out some of the more common drugs and routes of administration in Table 6, page 256.)

When taking chemotherapy in tablet form, keep the following points in mind:

TAKE THE DRUGS EXACTLY AS PRESCRIBED. With oral chemotherapy agents it is very important not to miss any doses, and to stop the medication on the specified day. Missing doses or prolonging the course can alter the drug's effect on the tumor and the side effects, particularly the effect on your blood count.

SIDE EFFECTS ARE USUALLY DELAYED BY A FEW HOURS. Most chemotherapy drugs taken by mouth produce side effects (for example, nausea) several hours after you take them. So plan accordingly and have antinauseants ready if you need them.

NEVER CARRY THE TABLETS AROUND IN AN UNLABELED CONTAINER OR MIXED WITH OTHER TABLETS. Some people like to carry around a few days' supply of all their medications in a plastic bag. This is flirting with disaster. Firstly, because they might take the wrong tablet at the wrong time and, secondly, because if they happen to fall ill (for example, with a fever due to low white cell count, related to the chemotherapy) any doctor or nurse looking after them would not know what drugs they are on, or even that they were on chemotherapy.

For intravenous injections and infusions, there is a different list of concerns. For these your veins are very important.

As you may have noticed, veins are variable, and they vary widely from person to person. Some people have large visible veins just under the skin, while others seem to have thin veins deep under the skin that seem even less prominent in an arm that is fat or swollen. Intravenous injections, as well as blood tests, may be more difficult in these latter people.

Furthermore, several of the chemotherapy drugs are very irritating to the walls of veins, and after repeated injections may cause the vein wall to become swollen and the vein to block completely.

For any or all of these reasons, some people will have veins that are (or become) quite difficult for the chemotherapy team to get into. The injections may become very uncomfortable and even painful. If the vein has clotted as a result of previous injections, they may become impossible to access.

If that happens—if venous access is no longer possible or comfortable—there are several different solutions that can give you, "synthetic veins" and provide access for the medications.

Here I'll give you a general description of some of the venous access systems, so that if you ever do require one of these, you will have some idea of what to expect.

There are two main kinds: with or without a reservoir.

SYSTEMS WITH A RESERVOIR (PORT-A-CATH® AND OTHER TYPES). Putting in a reservoir system is nowadays a simple standard procedure. It is usually done under a general anesthetic, though it can be done with a local anesthetic. The whole system is implanted under your skin so that nothing is actually above the surface. As one patient put it, "There's nothing hanging out of me."

A slim plastic catheter is put into a convenient vein, usually the one deep under your collarbone. It is then connected to a special reservoir about the size of a small walnut which is placed under the skin on your chest, usually near the collarbone.

This reservoir is covered with a special plastic membrane that can be penetrated, without damage, by a special needle that can be put into it through the skin. This is called a *Huber needle,* and no other type of needle should ever be used with the reservoir since it might damage the membrane. Putting the needle into the reservoir involves firm pressure but causes very little pain. Once the needle is in, fluids, drugs, and anything else you need intravenously (for instance blood, platelets, or antibiotics) can be given easily. At the end of the injection or infusion, the whole system is flushed with a small amount of saline containing an anticoagulant (heparin) to stop it clotting. And that's all there is to it.

The reservoir system needs to be flushed regularly (usually every few weeks or so) and can stay where it is indefinitely. Most of my patients with reservoir devices have no problems wearing clothing, even swimsuits. There is no cosmetic effect of the subcutaneous reservoir that can be detected easily, except by feeling it!

SYSTEMS WITHOUT A RESERVOIR (HICKMAN CATHETERS, PIC LINES, AND SIMILAR DEVICES). In certain situations, your doctor may recommend that you have a plastic tube (catheter) without a subcutaneous reservoir. In this situation, you will have a plastic tube emerging from the skin. The tube needs special care to make sure it does not collect bacteria.

The most common type of catheter used is the Hickman, and the advantage of a Hickman as opposed to a reservoir system is that it is possible to give larger amounts of fluids or transfusions quickly. So your doctor may recommend a Hickman catheter for you if you're likely to need several transfusions or large amounts of fluid at various stages of your treatment. The procedure to put in a system without a reservoir is almost the same as with the reservoir, except that at the end you will have a short length of plastic tube which is usually stored, curled up under a dressing, on the upper part of your chest.

There are quite a lot of "dos and don'ts" in caring for a Hickman and your chemotherapy or nursing team will show you how to do things if you want to participate. Some patients feel very good about participating in the care of their Hickman, and other patients prefer not to touch the catheter and let the nursing team do it all. Either approach is permissible!

And, finally, apart from tablets and intravenous injections, there are a few other routes used to administer chemotherapy drugs.

In some (rare and unusual situations), some chemotherapy drugs can be given directly into an artery supplying the tumor area, after a special catheter has been placed there. This method of administration is still being investigated in several tumors and it is not yet certain whether or not this is a more effective means of administration.

Other drugs can be given into an area of the body, such as the abdomen or the chest cavity. For example the drug bleomycin can be given when there is fluid in one of the areas to try to control the reaccumulation of the fluid.

In other special circumstances, some drugs can be given into the fluid that circulates over the brain and spinal cord (the CSF). This is called the *intrathecal* route of administration and it is used to prevent the spread of malignant cells to the brain and spinal cord in childhood leukemia, some lymphomas, and some other tumors, and is also used to treat secondaries if they are already there in certain cancers.

"What Side Effects Can I Expect?"

Almost all chemotherapy drugs (but not hormone treatments) cause some of these side effects: nausea and vomiting; suppression of the blood count, with potential susceptibility to infections, bruising, or anemia; hair loss, temporary; fatigue and exhaustion.

A few chemotherapy drugs, such as vincristine, do not cause these particular effects, but most of the others may, so it is worthwhile knowing a little bit about them.

Side Effects That Happen with Most Chemotherapy Drugs

FATIGUE AND EXHAUSTION. Most chemotherapy treatments may make you feel tired. The most marked tiredness largely begins to improve three or four weeks after the end of chemotherapy, but the improvement continues slowly over a long time. It is quite usual for people to feel noticeably less energetic than they did before the treatment for several months.

NAUSEA. For reasons that we do not understand, most chemotherapy drugs happen to affect a small center in the brain which is responsible for nausea and vomiting. This area is called the *chemotactic trigger zone*, or CTZ. It is not known why almost all chemotherapy drugs happen to stimulate this area, since they are so different in so many other respects. Nevertheless, they do, and as you can see in Table 7, page 257, some chemotherapy drugs are more likely to do it that others.

Time of Occurrence of Nausea

Nausea caused by chemotherapy generally depends to a certain extent not just on the drug, but also on the dose and how it is given—as a single "push" injection or as a long intravenous infusion, for example.

Nausea usually begins a few hours after the drugs have been given. Three to six hours is typical, though it is less for a few drugs. The most severe nausea usually continues for up to twenty-four or forty-eight hours. Typically, it is gone by the second or third day—in many cases, before that—though you may find that your appetite is poor for a day or so after that. Very often the nausea comes and goes in episodes. You may have no nausea at all in the middle of the second day, let's say, but then have a couple of hours when you feel somewhat nauseated again that evening.

Anticipatory Nausea

Many patients find that the nausea begins earlier with each course of chemotherapy. This is often due to *conditioning*, by which a response is created in which your behavior is changed by the strong stimulus of the treatment. So you may come to associate the sight of the hospital, for example, with nausea, and you might feel nauseated when the hospital first comes into view. You might even feel nausea when you encounter the name of the hospital. Some of my patients have told me that they experience nausea when they walk past the bus stop they usually use to go to the hospital. And one patient even retched at the sound of my voice when I telephoned her unexpectedly a year after therapy. (You have to believe me when I say that most of my patients do not usually retch at the sound of my voice!)

This type of conditioning is called *anticipatory nausea* and is quite common. In fact, about one-third of all patients on chemotherapy may experience it. If it does happen to you, it is important to realize that it is very common, and is not a sign that you're going mad. And it can be helped by starting your antinauseants (with a drug such as lorazepam) the night before your treatment.

Scapegoating

Some patients experience another form of conditioning with foods that they eat after the treatment. If you eat ravioli in the first few hours after chemotherapy, after some weeks you may find that every time you eat ravioli you feel nauseated. It is therefore worthwhile trying not to eat your favorite foods after your chemotherapy. In fact, some research showed that you can transfer this conditioned response of nausea onto a "scapegoat" food by eating it immediately after the chemotherapy. In the research, the scapegoat food was halva, a sweet paste made of pistachios which is available almost everywhere but which few people eat regularly. I recommend this trick to my patients, and many of them have found that they can use an unaccustomed food like that to deal with hunger after the chemotherapy but still avoid transferring the conditioned nausea onto their favorite foods.

Treatment of the Nausea Caused by Chemotherapy

The good news is that in the last few years there have been considerable advances in the treatment and control of nausea, so that nowadays a very high proportion of patients on even the most nausea-producing chemotherapy drugs have a relatively small number of episodes of vomiting, and many have no vomiting at all.

There are many different drugs that can be used to help you with nausea. They can be given in tablet form, by injections (with or before your chemotherapy), or by suppository. Suppositories are particularly useful if the nausea is bad, because they can be used when you are unable to keep tablets down, and also because the drug in the suppository is absorbed steadily over a period of hours.

There are several different types of antinauseants, and drugs from different groups can be used together. One particularly useful group of drugs have been introduced in the last two or three years. They are called H$_3$ blockers, a technical term that refers to the way they work, of which the most well known are ondansetron (Zofran) and granisteron (Kytril). If the nausea is bad and does not improve with the standard drugs, these can be effective.

For reasons that we do not yet understand these drugs work against chemotherapy-associated nausea in the first two or three days only and there is little value in taking them after that time.

Further Points about Antinauseant Medications

Table 8, page 259, gives you some idea of the range of drugs available to treat nausea, but bear in mind these points as well:

FIRST, YOU REALLY NEED TO TAKE THE CORRECT DOSES OF THE MEDICATIONS. Many people do not take enough of the drug, either taking too few tablets, or not taking them often enough, or both.

SECOND, IF YOU ARE HAVING DIFFICULTY KEEPING THE TABLETS DOWN, TALK TO YOUR DOCTOR. It might be worth considering suppositories.

THIRD, CHEMOTHERAPY-INDUCED NAUSEA GENERALLY IS SLIGHTLY WORSE IN THE MORNING. It is often helpful to keep an antinauseant tablet on your bedside table to take first thing in the morning, even before you get up.

Hair Loss (Alopecia)

Because chemotherapy drugs attack cells that are growing, and because the cells in the roots (follicles) of your hair are growing, many chemotherapy drugs will cause hair loss, *which is always temporary*. Your hair will grow back after the therapy is over.

The drugs usually affect the hair on your head more than they affect armpit, body, and pubic hair. But some drugs, Taxol for example, can affect all hair, including eyebrows.

Table 9 on page 262 shows which chemotherapy drugs are least and most likely to cause hair loss.

"When Does It Start?"

If your chemotherapy drugs are likely to cause hair loss, you will start noticing the loss in about three to four weeks. Usually the hair loss proceeds quite fast after that, and in some patients it can be complete in a few days. In others, the loss continues steadily over several weeks. If you have not had significant hair loss by about three months, that generally means it will not happen.

The secret of coping with this is to be prepared. That means going to look at some wigs even before you start the therapy. Your nursing team or social services team can usually supply information about this. It may be worth actually picking out a wig, though not necessarily buying it, so that you know it's there if it is needed.

A lot of my patients with long hair buy wigs with short hair. They tell me that not only do they get compliments on changing their hair style—most wigs are virtually undetectable these days—but also as their own hair regrows, they can stop wearing the wig after a short time.

Hair regrowth begins before the end of therapy, usually at about three or four months. Regrowth reaches a stage where you can do without a wig by about six to nine months or so. In general, the hair that regrows is softer and curlier, and in some cases it is darker too.

In a few situations it is possible to reduce the amount of hair loss, and sometimes prevent it altogether by using scalp cooling. This involves putting a cap which has been cooled in a refrigerator onto the head. It needs to be in position for about ten minutes before the chemo, and to remain in place for about ten minutes afterwards. It only works for those drugs that are excreted out of the bloodstream quickly—drugs such as Adriamycin. If the drug stays in the bloodstream for a long time—such as cyclophosphamide—then a cold cap will not prevent hair loss.

Infections
Chemotherapy affects your bone marrow. The most important and common problem is that chemotherapy can reduce the number of white cells in your blood and, therefore, your ability to fight infections.

The time of greatest risk generally begins about seven to ten days after chemotherapy. If the white cells are very low they sometimes may stay low until three weeks or so after that treatment. During that period, you may be particularly prone to getting an infection. The common infections are chest infections (with cough and green sputum), and throat infections (with a sore throat and pain on swallowing), but you may get a generalized infection with severe chills, shivering, and fever, without any particular problems detectable in the chest. It is also possible to get skin infections such as boils, or infections around the anus. Some people get urinary tract infections, passing urine frequently, with pain on passing the urine, sometimes with pain in the loin region round the lower back near the ribs.

The important thing here is to take your temperature if you feel ill, and particularly if you feel feverish or have shivers. If your temperature is more than 37.5°C on two occasions or more than 38°C once, then contact your doctor. If you have an infection while your white cells are low then it may be difficult for your body to deal with it. You may require antibiotics. These can be given by mouth in some circumstances, or you may need to be admitted to hospital for a week or so, in order to receive intravenous antibiotics.

Anemia (insufficient hemoglobin or too few red cells)
Another result of the bone marrow's being affected by chemotherapy is that it may make too few red cells or too little hemoglobin and you may become, temporarily, anemic. With anemia, you may look pale and feel tired and perhaps short of breath and weak. If those symptoms are severe, your doctor may decide that you need a blood transfusion.

Bruising and Bleeding
The *platelets* are the other factor manufactured in the marrow. They may also be reduced in number when the marrow is suppressed by chemotherapy. If that happens you may get little pinhead-sized purple spots—like tiny bruises, which is what they are—in the skin. These are called *petechiae* and you are most likely to see them on the shins. You may also get bleeding from the gums or the nose. Another possibility

is bleeding in the digestive tract, which may cause you to bring up blood or coffee-ground-like material or to pass jet-black stool. Another possibility is large bruises within the skin. If you get any of these problems, tell your doctor, who may want to check your platelets and, if they are very low, give you a transfusion of platelets.

Precautions Against Infection

While on chemotherapy there are several useful and practical things that you can do to decrease the chance of your getting an infection.

Be particularly careful about *washing your hands* after shaking hands with other people, going to the bathroom, or touching flat surfaces or door handles. While you are on chemotherapy, *never* touch your mouth or nose or eyes, or eat with your fingers until you have *washed your hands*.

Don't spend time with people who clearly have colds, flu or other infections.

Don't have dental work until you have discussed it with your oncologist and she or he has done a blood test or told you it is safe to have the work done.

If you are given prophylactic antibiotics, take them *exactly* as prescribed.

Problems with Appetite and Taste

Both appetite and the sense of taste can be affected by chemotherapy, sometimes to a marked extent. Your appetite may remain low for weeks or months at a time, and you may find that food tastes funny. Often patients describe it as a metallic sort of taste. These are difficult symptoms to deal with. It is generally worth trying out foods that you think might appeal to you, and "grazing," eating in smaller quantities but quite frequently. If you continue to lose weight due to eating too little, you can add high-protein and high-carbohydrate supplements. These are usually liquids or puddings and your dietitian can advise you what to do. There are quite a few instant breakfast mixtures which you can buy at the supermarket that work well too. If nothing helps, your doctor may recommend certain medications such as Provera which may increase appetite.

Does a Special Diet Help?

I've put this question in here because so many of my patients ask it. We hear so much about diet, and also about the fact that people with major dietary deficiencies (usually in other parts of the world) may become anemic, that it would seem logical that if you take extra care with your diet, the effects of chemotherapy might be reduced. Yet this is not the case.

In fact, provided your diet was reasonable and normal before the chemotherapy, there is nothing you need to do to it during therapy. The extent to which the chemotherapy affects the bone marrow is partly dependent on the way your body handles and excretes the drugs, and partly on the sensitivity of your bone marrow to the drugs (which in turn depends on things like your age, the amount of chemotherapy you have had previously, and so on). So if it happens that your bone marrow is greatly or easily affected by the chemotherapy, you need not think that this is your fault, or that there is something you should be doing (or eating) to prevent it.

Side Effects That Happen only with Particular Chemotherapy Drugs

Apart from the side effects mentioned above, there are a few others that are relatively common. I have set most of them out in Table 10 on page 262, not to alarm you or have you phoning your medical team, but so that you are aware of what may sometimes happen, and won't panic if it happens to you. Most of these disappear by themselves.

High-Dose Therapy with Bone Marrow Rescue, Bone Marrow Transplant, or Stem Cell Rescue

In a few of the cancers, better results can be achieved by giving very large doses of chemotherapy—doses that would normally kill you by destroying the bone marrow—and then "rescuing" you by giving back either your bone marrow or certain cells from your blood that were removed and stored before the chemotherapy was given. *High-dose therapy*, with stem cell or bone marrow rescue, has been shown to be effective in a small number of cancers—notably lymphomas, leukemias, recurrent Hodgkin's disease, and a few others.

In treating certain types of cancers, one of the major problems is that the drugs affect the patient's normal tissues, and very often the maximum amount of drug that can be given is limited because of the damage it will do to one part of the body or another. The tissue or organ that is most profoundly affected by a chemotherapy drug is called the *dose-limiting organ*, and with most chemotherapy drugs it is the bone marrow. Over the last twenty years, some ways have been devised to give higher doses of chemotherapy. Many of these techniques have proved very effective in certain cancers—we've mentioned the leukemias, some of the lymphomas, and certain cases of Hodgkin's disease—but so far they have not made a major contribution to the treatment of the more common cancers—such as cancers of the lung, breast, ovary, or bowel.

There are three basic high-dose procedures:

FIRST, BONE MARROW TRANSPLANT (BMT) is used where there is a primary cancer in the bone marrow: in practice that means basically leukemia or certain other similar conditions. The important thing is to find a relative, or someone on a marrow registry, who has a bone marrow that is genetically very similar to the patient. A proportion (less than 10 percent) of the marrow is collected from the donor. This involves a general anesthetic and multiple samples of marrow taken from the donor's pelvis.

Then the cancer patient is given high-dose chemotherapy, with or without radiotherapy. The dose of treatment is very high and is intended to kill all of the cancer cells. Of course, it would also kill the patient if he or she were not *rescued* (which is the actual medical term) by the marrow from the donor.

When the chemotherapy drug has been excreted by the patient, the marrow from the donor is given as a transfusion into a vein. After several days to a couple of weeks, the new bone marrow *takes*, the medical term for establishes itself, and begins to manufacture red cells, white cells, and platelets for the patient. The patient will usually have to take medications for a long time (perhaps indefinitely) to prevent the new marrow from rejecting the patient. This is called *graft-versus-host-disease* (GVHD). You're used to hearing about a body rejecting foreign tissue, but in this case it's the marrow that would do the rejecting. This type of therapy is now the standard therapy for certain types of leukemia (particularly acute myeloid leukemia) and some lymphomas, as long as there is a suitable donor available.

SECOND, AUTOLOGOUS BONE MARROW TRANSPLANT (ABMT), also called *high-dose treatment with bone marrow rescue*. In ABMT, the procedure is basically the same as the one I described for BMT, except that the patient is his or her own donor. The sample of marrow is collected from the patient, and then carefully preserved in a deep freeze. The patient then gets high-dose therapy of some description, and when the drugs have been excreted, the marrow is given back, again as a transfusion into a vein. This technique has also been useful in certain kinds of lymphoma and Hodgkin's disease, and in one or two other cancers as well. Presently, however, when the cancer originates in the breast, lung, ovary, or some other sites that have been studied, the high-dose treatment does not manage to kill all the cancer cells.

THIRD, STEM CELL RESCUE. In the last few years, we've discovered that instead of cells from the bone marrow, certain types of cells from the bloodstream will do the job just as well. Stem cell rescue usually involves collecting certain types of white cells from the bloodstream of the patient after he or she has been given medications to enhance the number of those cells. This is called *pheresis* and is usually done using two intravenous lines. The blood comes out of one line, goes into a centrifuge, a machine which skims off the desired cells, and is then returned to the patient via the other line. This type of treatment is not available everywhere, but is proving to be useful.

"What Are the Long Term Effects?"

INFERTILITY: Like radiation therapy, many kinds of chemotherapy may cause infertility in both males and females, meaning that the patient will be infertile and unable to produce or bear children.

Sometimes, there are measures that can be used to prevent infertility or to get around it (such as sperm banking) but this may not be possible in some cases. Also infertility is sometimes produced before treatment by the disease process itself.

SECOND MALIGNANCIES: With some types of chemotherapy—and in some cancers—there is an increased chance of developing a second type of cancer later.

Generally, this is more likely to happen when the original cancer was a lymphoma, but it can also happen very occasionally with other types of cancer, such as cancer of the breast. This is obviously a very serious long term effect, but fortunately it is very rare.

Biological Agents

Biological therapy is in its infancy but growing nicely. It has developed over the last twenty years and in the next decade it is expected to develop into a series of powerful weapons against cancer cells, perhaps to be used in treatment or perhaps to be used in prevention.

"How Do Biological Agents Work?"

Biological agents, originally called *biological response modifiers*, are complex and specific substances that mimic or interfere with the action of chemical triggers, used by cancer cells to keep themselves growing and reproducing, to provide themselves with a blood supply, and many other vital functions.

In other words, biological agents are "smart bombs" that home in specifically on key switches and control mechanisms in (or on) the cancer cells, and so destroy the cancer cells' ability to grow freely. By being specific to the control mechanisms used by cancer cells, they do not interfere (very much) with the normal growth and multiplication processes of normal cells. So their side effects are usually less sweeping.

They change the way the body reacts to cancer cells: they change the biological "atmosphere" inside the body and/or change the way that the body's defenses respond to cancer cells, and thus they affect the ability of cancer cells to grow or even survive. In other words, biologic agents don't attack every growing cell—as chemotherapy agents do—but rather they interfere with specific aspects and factors that support the growth of certain cancers. When these supports are removed or blocked or interfered with, the cancer cells find it very difficult to establish themselves and may fail and die, or simply be blocked from flourishing.

This is a new and vitally important avenue of investigation. But the first types of therapy that were tested for this purpose were treatments that changed the levels of various hormones in the body. By definition, really, earlier hormone treatments were the first types of biologic therapy.

For that reason, I'll briefly describe them first so that you understand the fundamental principles and the way they differ from chemotherapy, though the two are very often used together.

Hormone Therapy–Early Types of Biological Therapy

Some cancers depend on certain hormones that are present in the body. You can almost think of them as being fed and nurtured by those hormones. These cancers are often called *hormone-dependent* or *hormone-sensitive cancers*.

We have known for many decades that in many of these cancers, a change in the hormone levels can actually cause the cancer to shrink, often by a considerable amount. That is true of some cancers of the prostate and some cancers of the breast.

A high proportion of cancers of the prostate depend on the male hormone testosterone to grow. When the supply of testosterone disappears (as happens after castration) or the production of testosterone is interfered with by drugs (such as estrogens in the early days, and later with hormone-altering drugs such as cyproterone or fluanxol), the cancers are likely to shrink.

In breast cancer, the situation is similar. Many breast cancers, just over half in fact, are hormone sensitive. A test can be done on breast cancer cells in a biopsy to show whether or not they have receptors for hormones. If they do, then there is a very good chance that the cancer will respond to hormone treatment. When these breast cancers are deprived of a hormone—in this case, the female hormone estrogen—or are prevented from being able to use it, there is a high chance that they will stop growing or actually shrink.

The hormone environment can be changed by removing the ovaries, or by interfering either with the production of estrogen (as the drugs that inhibit an enzyme called *aromatase* do) or with its ability to bind onto the cancer cell (this latter is what tamoxifen and similar drugs do).

Now, here is one of the most important features about hormone treatments. Their mechanism of action is to change the internal hormonal climate and produce a new climate that makes it very difficult for cancer cells to grow and spread. So hormonal therapies—including well known medications such as tamoxifen, for example—*do not attack every growing cell*.

And that highlights the difference between chemotherapy agents which are fundamentally undiscriminating in their ability to damage growing cells (although most of them have been selected to do much more damage to cancer cells than to normal cells), and hormone agents which specifically interfere with something that the cancer cells need for success.

That is the basic principle by which hormonal agents work. And the same principle underlines all of the biologic response modifier treatments—now abbreviated to *biologics*—which take the same idea much further.

Biological Therapy ("Biologics") as Treatment of Cancer

For the last fifty years or more cancer researchers have been looking much more specifically at the things that cancer cells need in order to establish themselves and spread.

We have made great strides in that research (although of course there is much further to go) and we now know *some* of the things that some cancers depend on in order to flourish. If—so the logic goes—we can interfere with these factors, then we can cut off the cancer's ability to grow, exactly as an air force can interfere with an army by bombing its supply roads, rails, and fuel depots.

The research into biologic agents really consists of two processes:

FIRST, identify something that cancer cells depend on—a *target molecule*;

SECOND, produce a specific agent (a smart bomb to follow the air force analogy) that interferes with the cancer cell's ability to use that target molecule effectively.

Researchers have been looking for such smart bombs for decades and as far back as the late 1970s had produced specific antibodies that recognize and bind to certain molecular targets (called *antigens*) on the surface of cancer cells. Then, they hoped to find a large number of these which could be detected on the surface of cancer cells, preferably on the surface of all cancer cells, and not on the surface of normal cells.

By the early 1970s techniques had been perfected that allowed scientists to tailor-make protein antibodies of a single pure kind (called *monoclonal antibodies*) which bind to specific antigens.

Monoclonal antibodies are pure single antibodies produced in the laboratory to react against a single target (as opposed to the natural action of our bodies which produce dozens of antibodies against, for example, the flu virus). When they were first invented it was hoped that they would become true magic bullets, capable of carrying poisons or radioactive isotopes directly onto the targeted cancer cells, and avoiding normal cells.

This groundbreaking research was the beginning of the creation of biological smart bombs and was initially used to bind to antigens found on the surface of certain kinds of lymphoma.

Furthermore, these monoclonal antibodies could be "armed" with a sort of "tail"—which could be a radioactive isotope, or a poison, or a chemotherapy drug—and thus therapy could be guided exclusively to cancer cells and away from any normal cells.

A few initial successes led to the hope that all cancers might have antigens which could be treated in that way. That didn't happen, but the idea triggered a whole new avenue of research which is currently making great strides.

The Current Generation of Molecular Targets

What's been going on in the last decade or so in the area of biologic therapy is both exciting and promising.

Research has been directed to identifying particular types of molecular targets on the surface of cancer cells, not simply by their presence—meaning their presence on cancers and their absence from normal cells—but on their function. The search has been for molecules that cancer cells use and depend on, and that normal cells do not. In other words, researchers have been looking for molecules on the cancer cells that actually *do something* for the cancer. If you'll allow me a crude analogy, it's like trying to arrest terrorists by looking at the clothing worn by a crowd of people. You might find, let's say, that when you select everyone who is wearing a black beret you haul in a lot of terrorists but a lot of civilian bystanders as well, and many of the terrorists seem to escape. If on the other hand you haul in all the people who are carrying bullet-clips around their waists then you (probably!) won't pull in any civilians—because carrying a bullet-clip is something that armed terrorists do, and civilians don't.

The situation is similar with cancer cells. Until the 1980s, our research was really only capable mostly of identifying the items of clothing. In the last two decades, research his been unearthing molecules that have a *function* for the cancer cell (like the bullet-clip in the analogy). And *that* has opened up a vast new area of exploration.

For example, early in this research, it was shown that some cancers had a special type of "on switch" by which they could be stimulated and activated. This switch was turned on by a hormone called *epidermal growth factor* (EGF). When a particular cancer possessed the receptors for EGF then it usually turned out to be more aggressive than average.

Further research led to the development of specific monoclonal antibodies that could bind to the EGF receptor, and when they did that they blocked it so that the cancer cells could not be activated by EGF. (Just as, let's say, a clever criminal might be able to produce a key that fitted into a lock but if the key broke off and jammed in the lock, that door could never be used.)

The sequence of events is practical proof that this kind of focused research really works. First, researchers identified the molecular target on the more aggressive breast cancers (comparable to spotting the lock-plates around the actual locks). The target was named *her2/neu*, and then it was found that it was the lock that was activated by EGF. Then the antibody was produced—with a great deal of brilliant and concentrated research by Dr. Dennis Slamon's group—and it was named *trastuzumab*. (The names are notoriously difficult to pronounce, but when they end in *-mab* that generally denotes the fact that they are monoclonal antibodies. And because trastuzumab binds to a molecule called a *receptor*, by the name of *her2/neu*, when it was produced commercially it was called *Herceptin*.)

The Herceptin story is a perfect example of how a sequence of consecutive discoveries led to a drug that is now used in the treatment of a particular type of cancer (in this case, breast cancer). Herceptin has been called, not inappropriately, "the poster child of the biologics." And you can see why.

So, the whole point about the biologics is that they are specific and selective. They attack particular molecular sites—one type of lock, in our analogy—whereas chemotherapy agents attack all growing cells. In other words, biologic therapy is really a modern incarnation of the magic bullet, the weapon that homes in on the bad guys and has little or no effect on the normal good guys.

Other Biologics

Interferons are biologics produced by the immune system during acute infections (such as flu). Early studies showed that interferons were active against various types of cancer cells. Many years of clinical studies have now shown that interferons are useful, but only in certain types of cancer. They are most valuable in the treatment of Kaposi's sarcoma. They were once useful in the treatment of hairy-cell leukemia but have now been replaced by something better.

The *interleukins* are a group of substances, produced by cells in the body that act as signals between cells. We do not fully understand all of the things that interleukins do, but one of them is to activate or "arm" certain types of cells in the immune system. It was initially hoped that by giving large amounts of a certain interleukin—interleukin-2 or IL-2—specific cells in the immune system would be able to obliterate cancer cells. The early results were very exciting. Certainly, the treatment was somewhat unpleasant and rather hazardous, but there was no question that responses were seen.

Later, it was shown that better results could be achieved by separating those immune cells from the bloodstream and then treating them with IL-2 in the laboratory. Those cells were then called *lymphokine activated killer* (LAK) cells. With further studies, it seems that the effects of IL-2 or LAK cells are most pronounced and most useful in kidney cancer (renal-cell carcinoma) and melanoma.

It has always been something of a mystery that a cancer could spread to a lymph node and that inside that lymph node the cancer cells and the lymphocytes could apparently live next to each other in peaceful coexistence. Researchers separated lymphocytes from areas of tumor and demonstrated that, once separated, those lymphocytes showed certain kinds of activity against cancer cells. It is presumed that, somehow, this anticancer activity is not sufficient to stop the cancer cells, or that perhaps the cancer cells produce something that neutralizes or paralyzes the natural activity of those lymphocytes. The use of cells separated from a tumor—thus called *tumor infiltrating lymphocytes* (TIL)—was investigated and although they are interesting, they may not have a major role in the treatment of most cancers.

There are several other substances that the body may produce in response to certain conditions—including cancer—that might be used in treatment. For example, there is a substance called *tumor necrosis factor* (TNF) which initially showed great promise in the treatment of ovarian cancer that had spread around the abdomen. Investigations and clinical trials are going on with several substances like this, and one or several of them may have a defined role in cancer treatment in the future.

Biological Therapy as an Adjunct to Other Cancer Treatments

Some biologics are useful in stimulating the growth of normal cells (particularly bone marrow cells) when they have been damaged by chemotherapy. For example *colony-stimulating factors* (CSFs) are substances produced in the bone marrow which stimulate the marrow into increasing and speeding up its production of cells. When the marrow has been seriously affected by chemotherapy—and the patient has life-threatening infections, severe anemia, or bleeding—CSFs can speed up recovery. The CSFs have different names, such as G-CSF and GM-CSF (a commercial brand is Neupogen) depending on which cells in the marrow they stimulate. The one that stimulates red cells is called *erythropoietin*, usually abbreviated to EPO.

Due to considerable advances in techniques, CSFs can now be produced in large quantities. Their use with chemotherapy has shown that they do reduce the period of very low white cells. However, they are used only when the consequences of marrow suppression are very severe (for example, life-threatening infections) and where it is clear that proceeding with chemotherapy will make a major difference (such as achieving a cure or prolonged remission). So they are not routinely used in every case in which chemotherapy has reduced white or red cells or platelets. (Table II, page 264, lists some of the current generation of biologics.)

"What Is a Clinical Trial–And Should I Go into One?"

This section of Part Two explains the whole idea of clinical trials—why they are important, how they have contributed to advances in cancer treatment, why they improve the standards of care, and why it's really important that you at least consider seriously the idea of entering one.

As one of my patients said, quite gently, to me, "To put it mildly, doctor, the treatment of most cancers these days is less than satisfactory." She was right.

About half of all the patients diagnosed with a cancer this year will be cured. For those people, most of the cures will be achieved by surgery, together with radiotherapy and chemotherapy in some cases. For a small number of cancers, cure is most likely to be achieved by chemotherapy.

It is fair (but a generalization) to say that in all those cases, the treatment is by and large satisfactory. But there is continued and very active research going on to make the treatment even more effective and to reduce the side effects as far as possible.

In most of the other cases, we, in the medical profession, are still trying to find out the best method of treatment. So when cure is possible, we are trying to improve the treatment and decrease its side effects, and when cure is not possible we are trying to work out the most effective treatment. That means that we have to do careful and detailed and painstaking research—and the system by which this done is called a *clinical trial*.

Usually in cancer treatment we have to undertake a detailed and careful comparison of one treatment, which we believe might be an improvement, with the standard treatment. This is usually done by means of what is called a clinical trial. The word *trial* is used to mean that the new treatment is being tried against the old—not that the patient (or the doctor) is being tried!

In order to remove any bias that may come from a doctor (who may believe that he or she already knows the answer) or a patient, the participants are entered into the trial by randomization. That means that whether you get the standard treatment or the newer treatment is decided randomly by a computer off in some central office. That sounds impersonal, but it is the only way to make sure that the trial results are valid. Imagine what would happen if a doctor believed that treatment X was better than treatment Y. He or she might put all the patients expected to do well (say, the younger patients with smaller tumors) on treatment X, and put the older and iller ones on treatment Y. The trial might then show that patients of treatment X did fare better than those on treatment Y. But it would not be because of the treatment, it would be because of the way the patients for each treatment were selected. So randomization—computer coin-flipping, really—is the only way to make sure that the trial yields results that are believable.

Furthermore, if during its progress a trial shows that one treatment really is dramatically better than the other, then the trial will be stopped and everyone will receive the better treatment. This is not likely to happen unless the results are truly impressive. (It happened recently with the addition of the drug Herceptin to chemotherapy as adjuvant therapy after surgery for breast cancer.) But it is important that you realize you will not be denied a miracle if one occurs.

Now, you might think, "If my doctor does not know what the best treatment is, surely he can't be much good anyway." Strangely enough, it's the exact opposite: medical centers that are involved in clinical trials actually produce better results than the average, even for those patients who not enrolled in clinical trials. In other words, doctors actively trying to find out answers in cancer treatment are generally better at looking after their patients than doctors who do not. Several studies have shown that centers at which clinical trials are carried out have an overall higher standard of care than centers at which such trials are not being done. Presumably this is because the demands of organizing and running a trial keep standards up to a high level, and that causes a spin-off effect to the benefit of all patients, whether they are in clinical trials or not.

Finally, all clinical trials have to be reviewed and approved by the hospital or center's ethics committee. This means that there is no chance of anything dishonest or unethical happening, or of something that is unfair or prejudicial being done to you. You will be given a detailed consent form to sign (which will previously have been assessed in detail by the ethics committee) and you will be given a copy of it to keep. If for any reason, you cannot tolerate the treatment any more, or simply wish to stop being in the clinical trial, you have the right to leave. You just have to tell your doctor that that is what you wish. Obviously your doctor hopes that you will not to do that, but if you want to, you can, and the relationship with your doctor, and the care you receive, will not suffer as a result.

It's worth your while considering a clinical trial because clinical trials are the only way in which knowledge advances.

It was through clinical trials that the world learned about the benefits of the adjuvant treatment of breast cancer, the best treatment of childhood leukemia, and that bone marrow transplant did work for adult leukemia.

So trials are of major importance. But we have to face the fact that they are often awkward things to approach—for the doctor as well as the patient. The doctor has to talk about the limits of current knowledge, and you or your family may think the doctor is saying, "I don't know what to do." But a clinical trial is not a confession that a doctor doesn't know what treatment is best, it is a statement that the entire medical profession does not know which of two (or more) treatments being compared is better. We have to admit that we do not know the answers, and we are therefore asking your help in finding out what to do.

Many patients in clinical trials initially feel that they are, in some respects, guinea pigs. And to some extent, that is true. Until we know the best and definitive treatment of every cancer everyone will be a guinea pig. But in a clinical trial the world gains knowledge that is firm and believable. Clinical trials need a lot of work (on the part of the medical team) and they need a certain amount of cooperation from the patient's side, too. But at present, clinical trials are the only way to make true and credible progress against cancer.

Talking with Your Medical Team

One of my patients put it well when she said, in a thoughtful and philosophical tone, "It's not easy being a patient—you don't get any training for it, you don't know who everybody is or what they do, and you're not sure what's expected of you."

Her points are well taken.

As a new cancer patient, you are thrust into a situation that is unfamiliar, within a system that is complex and (sometimes) unintelligible, run by people whom you don't yet know. In addition, you have little idea of what you are either supposed to do or allowed to feel. All this is bad enough, but there is also the fact that you are obviously worried about what is happening to you and about your future, and you may also have physical symptoms. It is no wonder that you feel bewildered.

On occasions, too, you may find yourself becoming irritated, particularly if you have to repeat your story over and over again.

In this section, I am going to set out some simple guidelines to help you get to know the new faces, and give you some pointers about what the various team members do. Then I will describe some ways of approaching a few common situations: describing your symptoms, getting more information, and obtaining a second opinion.

Getting to Know Your Team Members

In an ideal world, all the members of your medical team would introduce themselves and explain what they do.

Unfortunately our world is frequently far from ideal, and clinics are full of highly specialized people under time pressure. How do you work out who's who and what's what?

"Who Are You and What Do You Do?"

The number of different people who you are likely to meet depends on what kind of tests and treatment are recommended in your case and what types of services are available at your cancer center.

Bear in mind these two important principles:

First, you are allowed to ask them to repeat their names if you didn't get them first time!

Second, you are allowed to ask which part of the team they work with! It's often worth having a little try, and placing them, and then asking for correction, "I'm sorry, I'm a bit confused—are you working with Dr. Smith or are you part of Dr. Brown's team?"

This way of asking is more pleasant than a rather brusque, "Who are you, and what do you do?" which may sound a little inquisitorial to someone who wasn't expecting it.

Here is a very simplified list of the people that you might meet, with just a word or two about some aspect you may not have considered:

FAMILY DOCTOR (GENERAL PRACTITIONER). With all the specialists and sub-specialists that you may be seeing, it's easy to downplay the importance of your GP. But it is *essential* that you have a GP and that all your clinic doctors know who it is so that copies of records and reports can be sent there, and your own doctor can be updated as to what's going on. So if you don't have a GP right now, please find one in the next week or so!

GENERAL SURGEON. Most cancers are likely to be diagnosed as a result of a biopsy by a general surgeon. It is important that you get a clear picture of what happens next and who does what. So make sure you write down the name of the person you are being referred to (if that is what happens) and his or her specialty.

ONCOLOGISTS. Oncologists are cancer doctors. There are three main settings in which oncologists work—academic centers, general hospitals, and in the community. By and large radiation oncologists are based in academic centers or large hospitals (because the radiotherapy machines are a major investment and are centralized), whereas medical oncologists can work in any of the three settings.

RADIATION ONCOLOGIST. Radiation oncologists are MDs who have training and experience in the cancers, with further training in the use of radiation. They work in very close collaboration with medical oncologists and surgeons, usually working in multidisciplinary clinics. They are in the best position to explain to you the overall plan for treatment if it includes radiation, and its potential side effects and benefits. Most have a subspecialty (e.g., breast cancer, lung cancer).

MEDICAL ONCOLOGIST. Medical oncologists are MDs who have training and experience in the cancers, with further training in the use of chemotherapy drugs (including hormone and biological treatment). They work in very close collaboration with radiation oncologists and surgeons. Many work in multidisciplinary clinics, though some are in community settings. They are in the best position to explain to you the overall plan for your treatment, if it includes chemotherapy or other drugs, and its various side effects and potential benefits. Many have a subspecialty.

SURGICAL ONCOLOGISTS. Many surgeons specialize in the treatment of cancer, and have considerable training and experience in the use of surgery. Their opinion is of great importance regarding whether an operation is required, and what the consequences would be. They tend to work in multidisciplinary units or clinics. They usually specialize in a particular cancer or group of cancers.

GYNECOLOGIC ONCOLOGISTS. These are gynecologic surgeons who have specialized in cancer surgery. NEUROSURGICAL ONCOLOGISTS are neurosurgeons who have specialized in cancer neurosurgery.

RADIATION TECHNOLOGISTS. These are the people who supervise all the details of your radiation treatment. If you are having radiation therapy you will get to know one or more of your radiation technologists very well—and they also form an additional vital link between you and the radiation oncologist. Similarly *radiation therapy planners* and *radiation physicists* may be involved in your treatment plan.

PRIMARY CARE NURSE OR CLINIC NURSE. Some nursing departments organize their nurses so that each patient has one identifiable primary care nurse who is the central and constant point. You will usually have a phone number for contact and questions.

CLINICAL NURSE SPECIALISTS. Clinical nurse specialists are nurses who have training and expertise in specific areas; for example, care of colostomies and ileostomies. (These nurses are often called *stoma nurses*.) Others have training and expertise in the administration of chemotherapy drugs or in the care of implanted devices for intravenous access (like the Port-a-Cath®). Other areas of specialization include clinical trials and pain control.

FELLOWS: A Fellow is an MD who is a specialist-in-training. She or he is in a training program (usually three years) in a particular area (medical oncology maybe, or gynecologic oncology). During that time the Fellow will rotate through several different areas to gain experience and training. That means that when you are seen by a Fellow in the clinic, you may only get to know him or her for a few months (three or so is usual, although up to a year is quite possible).

CLINICAL ASSOCIATES OR CLINICAL ASSISTANTS. These are MDS who work in a clinic but are not in training to be specialists. Many of them come from family medicine, though some are academics or have other interests in medicine. They are permanent members of the medical clinic staff.

PHARMACISTS. In cancer therapy, pharmacists are of enormous importance. They can explain exactly how to take your take-home medications, what side effects to look out for, and what problems require immediate assistance if they occur. They will give you information sheets on the drugs that you are taking, and it really is worth reading these sheets when you get home.

PHYSIOTHERAPISTS. These are extremely important at many stages of your treatment and particularly after surgery. (For example, they can help you remobilize or get your shoulder back to normal after breast surgery.)

SPEECH PATHOLOGISTS AND SPEECH THERAPISTS. These may be needed to help you to recover your speech (or learn new ways of speaking) after surgery to the larynx.

SOCIAL WORKERS. These are extremely important. They may be greatly helpful in dealing with all kinds of adjustments (including financial) and can help you by discussing the services available in your area.

CHAPLAINS. Nowadays, chaplaincy includes many different faiths and religions. Many cancer centers have chaplains in the Christian, Jewish, and Muslim religions. If you want to see a chaplain or religious counselor of a particular faith, ask a nurse or a social worker in your clinic whom to contact.

PATIENT ADVOCATE. The patient advocate (often called the *ombudsman*) is there to make sure your rights are not infringed. If things happen to go wrong between you and your medical team, the patient representative is responsible for investigating what you think what wrong, helping you find out the facts of the matter, and sorting out any remedy that is necessary and possible.

DIETICIANS. Often treatment (particularly chemotherapy, and certain kinds of surgery) affects your appetite and/or your ability to eat. A dietician can help you to discover more appetizing food and to eat in a healthier way. This can make a great deal of difference to how you feel.

PSYCHIATRISTS. These are MDS who specialize in mental health. Referral to a psychiatrist, if you are seriously depressed for example, can make a very big difference.

PSYCHOLOGISTS AND PSYCHOTHERAPISTS. These are not MDS, but they specialize in the support and psychotherapy ("talk therapy") of many of the effects of the cancers and their treatment. They usually will see you regularly (say once or twice a week) for discussions and may be of great assistance in helping you sort out what may be disturbing you and in reinforcing your own coping strategies to improve your quality of life.

SUPPORT GROUPS. Many cancer centers have their own support groups nowadays, and there are even greater numbers of support groups in the community. (You can ask the national organizations to give you a list of support groups in your area.) They are guided usually by a psychologist, or sometimes by a trained volunteer.

LIBRARIANS. Nowadays many cancer centers have a patient library with books (like this one!) written for the general public. Librarians can help you get more information (booklets, pamphlets and so on) and can steer you toward Web sites than are reliable and useful.

GENETIC COUNSELORS. The number of cancers in which an identifiable genetic abnormality is involved is still small, but growing. If there are several people in your family who have had breast cancer or ovarian cancer, for example, you may be referred for genetic testing. This may be of importance for your children (so that your daughters may be advised to start screening at an earlier age than average, for example, or to consider other forms of prevention).

It has often been said that medical care is like a high-stakes relay race, with your care being handed clearly from one person to another. You can help in that process by knowing a bit about who is meant to do what, and asking the right questions of the right people.

Talking about Your Symptoms

You will often be asked to describe your symptoms. To do this efficiently is actually quite difficult!

Here are a few pointers which may help:

FIRST, AS YOU DESCRIBE THE MEDICAL PROBLEM, BE FACTUAL. Some patients might exaggerate the pain or nausea in order to convince the doctor. They may feel that somehow this will produce better or more urgent therapy. On the other hand, some patients underplay their symptoms in order to appear stoic. You should ignore both of these temptations and try to describe your medical problems in as factual and neutral terms as you can. It's not easy, but if you do that, you will certainly end up with your doctor or nurse supporting you and being on your side. If you try to overplay or underplay your problems, there is a risk that they will feel alienated and will be less willing to help you. In an ideal world, that wouldn't happen. But you're a human being, and so are they, and it can! Play it straight. You don't need to convince your doctor of either the severity of your symptoms or of your own personal courage.

SECOND, USE YOUR OWN LANGUAGE. Just because your doctors or nurses use medical jargon, you don't need to. There's nothing wrong with using your own words to describe the problem. In fact, using jargon that you only partly understand might cause difficulties by giving the wrong slant to your problem.

THIRD, WHEN YOU'RE EMBARRASSED, DON'T HESITATE TO SAY SO! We all find certain kinds of medical symptoms and problems embarrassing. They're very often the kind of personal details we don't talk about to anyone else. So when you start talking about something that is embarrassing, just say so, "I'm sorry...this is embarrassing to talk about." Remember, emotions that are acknowledged are partly neutralized.

Asking for Information

When it comes to getting information from your medical team, your own feelings and fears may make it a bit difficult for you to ask the right questions and to remember the answers. Here are some tips:

FIRST, try to think of the most important questions before the discussion with your doctor.

SECOND, to help you remember the important points, write them down on a piece of paper that you can take with you.

THIRD, in addition to a written list, it's a good idea to take a friend or a relative with you. Often the other person can remember things that the doctor said but which you later forget, and can also often remember the questions you wanted to ask but haven't gotten round to yet. Every healthcare professional knows how difficult it is to understand and retain information when it is serious and when it is about you. So nowadays nobody will mind your using anything, such as a list and a friend, that helps you retain information and details.

FOURTH, remember that this consultation is not your only chance to ask questions. Of course, sometimes there won't be advance notice of an important subject. You may hear bad news quite unexpectedly, for example. But even then, there is always the next interview at which you can ask for clarification. And if you're not clear about what you've heard, don't hesitate to ask for clarification. Once your doctor or nurse has answered your questions, it's not a bad idea for you to recap that answer and say something like, "So you're saying that..." or, "If I've got that right, you mean that..." Such a comment makes it clear what you have understood, and often encourages your doctor or nurse to explain things clearly and intelligibly.

FIFTH, often, definitive answers are not possible. It's good if you can accept that uncertainties are common, particularly with questions about the future. When the conversation is about very serious matters that threaten your health or your view of the future, it's easy to imagine that your doctor or nurse knows what is going to happen but will not tell you. Usually, that's not the case. If a type of treatment has, let's say, a 40 percent chance of success, and therefore a 60 percent chance of failure, very often there is no way to predict which group you will be in.

It may help you get a grip on the situation if you can understand how progress will be measured: "So you'll decide from the X-rays if the treatment is working…" But with cancer therapy, there is often a lot of uncertainty. Uncertainty can be extremely unpleasant and difficult to cope with. But it exists, and it doesn't mean your doctor is holding out on you!

SIXTH, if you feel doubt or dissatisfaction with your healthcare team, or one member of it, try to express those doubts as diplomatically as you can. I say that not to save my own skin (or at least not *merely* to save my own skin) but to help you get better service. Most doctors and nurses, like all human beings, respond to constructive criticism well, and respond to destructive criticism either defensively or angrily. If you are able to voice your criticisms with a "tick what's right before you cross out what's wrong" balance, you'll find that you are much more likely to get your needs met.

Getting a Second Opinion
If you have any doubts about your medical situation, or if you do not fully understand what your doctor is saying, or even if you are not sure that his or her view of the situation is the only option, then a second opinion may be a great help to you.

Here, again, there are a couple of points to keep in mind:

First, it is very helpful to inform your doctor that you would like a second opinion. In fact, this is not merely a matter of etiquette and politeness, this is essential, because your doctor will need to send a summary or copies of your case-record to the second doctor. Without accurate details of your cancer, the tests that you have had, and any previous treatment, the second doctor will be unable to comment usefully. So do make sure you tell your first doctor that you would like a second.

Finally, if the second opinion is the same as the first, stop and think.

There is considerable temptation to shop around and see many doctors until you find one that says what you want to hear. Usually, that does not happen. Often, in fact, the act of seeing many doctors is really an expression of denial, part of a desire to reject the diagnosis or the view of the future. So if you hear the same thing from more than one doctor, think about what that means. Of course, some people will be deeply distressed by that. In those circumstances, it may be better to get help to reduce the distress (further discussion with your doctor, or counseling perhaps) rather than continue on what may turn out to be a deeply disappointing and frustrating quest.

"Isn't There an Easier Way?"

Complementary Medicine and Remedies

Another major problem triggered by that sense of dread associated with the word *cancer* is this: the greater the fear, the greater the urge to believe that all cancers can be quickly and easily cured, without side effects, by alternative, complementary, folk, or home remedies.

This creates the serious problem of raising false hopes. In this section I will discuss the whole area of complementary remedies, not because I want to be negative or officious about the facts, but because I think it is important that you do not get hurt or damaged by unrealistic expectations and wild hopes that are sometimes raised by people who sincerely believe they can achieve things that, in fact, they cannot.

As you'll see at the end of this section, there is an important take-home message: *what* you do may be less important than *how* you do it.

It may be less important *whether* or not you decide to try a complementary remedy (because so many people do try one or more of them) than *how* you do it. Are you pinning all your hopes on it, sacrificing your precious time, money, or energy on it, only to find—if it does not work—that you feel disappointed, depressed, and deserted, and regret your psychological investment?

The Fundamental Difference Between Conventional and Complementary Practices

Before I start discussing this very controversial topic, I should first clarify what I mean when I use the words *conventional* and *complementary*.

When I say *conventional physician* I mean a person who has been trained in a medical school, is licensed by the government, and is practicing medicine in a way that is approved by the regulatory boards in place. That's all I mean—*conventional medicine* is the regular, regulated practice of medicine.

By *complementary medicine*, I mean everything else. That includes anything that is given to or done to people who are ill (or perceive themselves to be ill) by someone who either is not a conventional physician, or is a conventional physician but is using unorthodox methods that are not conventionally used by his or her peers.

But there is more to it than that.

The difference between conventional and complementary medicine is not only a matter of licensing and regulation, it is also a matter of approach to truth and validity.

In conventional medicine, by and large, drugs and techniques are tested in a carefully designed way in an attempt to *disprove* their effectiveness. The drug or technique earns its place by being tested, in a clinical trial or research study, in a way by which an *ineffective* drug or technique would be demonstrated as such, and could then be discarded.

This principle is called *falsifiability*, meaning that the drug or technique has to "stand up or shut up." The ones that work are clearly shown to work and the ones that don't are out. That is the basis of all the clinical trials that are published (and often then reported in the media).

This principle of falsifiability underlies all of science (including physics, chemistry and everything else). The laws of nature and the hypotheses about the physical universe that we accept as true are those that have been tested in an attempt to falsify them, and have survived the attempt.

Now not everything that is used today in conventional medicine has been tested (yet). A lot of what conventional physicians have been doing for centuries has been adopted by custom and habit. But all *new* drugs and medications are tested. Everything used in the treatment of cancer, for example, has been tested in a trial designed on the "attempt to disprove" principle.

By contrast, complementary medicines have not been tested in that way. And most complementary medicine practitioners are adamant that they cannot and never will be. Despite that, there are a few remedies that originated as complementary medicines which have been subjected to proper testing. Most have been shown to be ineffective but there are four or five examples of remedies—including a Chinese herbal remedy for childhood eczema—that have proved effective in noncancerous conditions. These can legitimately be regarded as scientifically proven medications. But there are no complementary cancer remedies or techniques that have made the grade in that way.

Over the years, about a dozen potential anticancer complementary remedies have been formally tested in proper trials. But none of them has turned out to have any effect in any cancer. In other words, very few of the complementary remedies that are suggested for use in the treatment of a cancer have been properly tested, and of those that have been tested, none has been shown to work.

So with the definitions and results in mind, we can now go on to discuss the pluses and the minuses of complementary medicine.

Let's start by asking a very simple question: why does all this matter?

Why does it matter if somebody claims to be able to cure every type of cancer with an herbal remedy that has no side effects?

"So What's the Problem with Unfounded Claims?"

At first sight, it might appear that nobody is seriously harmed.

It might appear that overstatements, exaggerations and far reaching promises are certainly regrettable but, particularly because the media continuously bombards us with so much that is not quite true, a bit of overoptimism and overstatement cannot matter all that much.

I think it does matter.

In my own clinical experience time after time, I have seen people's hopes raised to high levels with false promises, only to be followed by serious and deep disappointment, even depression, often made worse by a feeling of having been exploited and cheated.

Undoubtedly, some of the problem is caused by the size of the perceived threat. When a threat is seen as very large, we are all more vulnerable and perhaps more gullible than we are during normal times. With an instantly emotive word like *cancer*, it is not surprising that the history of unfounded claims is centuries old and has attracted claimants (many of them totally sincere) from a wide variety of backgrounds.

The remedies hailed as the "cure for cancer" come from a wide variety of sources. Some are derived from folk remedies, some from ancient traditional medicines, and some are new discoveries or mixtures formulated by people outside conventional science and medicine.

The claims made in their support usually state that the remedy has produced cures that were not expected, or has prolonged the life of a person who was expected to die, backed up by dozens of testimonials from grateful patients. In the great majority of cases, the remedy or intervention is claimed to have very few side effects. Often it is noted that these claims have been rejected by conventional medical practitioners, sometimes followed up by persecution, and even prosecution, of the proponents of the complementary remedy healer.

Given the long history of such claims and the hundreds of hopes that were falsely raised and then disappointed in the past, there have also been equally strong counterclaims.

Furthermore it does sometimes happen—though not often—that the allure of a wonder-cure free of side effects is so strong that people with a curable cancer forsake the conventional treatment that is being recommended. (Cases like this are rare. But in my career I have been involved in the care of two patients with Hodgkin's disease, one with non-Hodgkin's lymphoma and one with seminoma—all of whom forsook their conventional therapy for complementary remedies which, sadly, had no effect on their cancers.)

The Upside of Complementary Medicine

Having underlined the danger of unfounded promises, however, let us now look at the benefits offered by complementary medicine and its practitioners—which are considerable.

Complementary medicine practitioners are generally better in the area of the doctor-patient relationship than many of their conventional medicine counterparts. In general, patients who visit a complementary medicine practitioner feel they are likely to get better communication and more empathy, in an atmosphere that is more conducive to discussing emotions. Patients are more likely to see the same practitioner each visit—seeing a different person each visit is a common problem with cancer centers—and the consultations are less likely to be rushed. While conventional physicians are perceived to be good at "disease-doctoring," complementary medicine practitioners are perceived as being better at "person-doctoring."

In addition, there are many philosophical attractions of complementary medicine and I have summarized these as follows:

Idea	What the Idea Means
THE CONCEPT OF HEALTH	Remedy or treatment not only conquers disease but establishes positive health
CONCEPT OF FORCE OR ENERGY	Basis is often a universal hypothesis of natural forces
UNIFYING HYPOTHESIS OF DISEASE	All diseases are caused by an imbalance or negative force(s)
SELF-HEALING	Forces are accessible within patient that can reverse course of disease
NATURAL	Inherent advantage of remedy is derived from natural products over synthetic
TRADITIONAL	Based on centuries of folk wisdom: knowledge that ancestors had that was lost
EXOTIC	Imported from different culture—previously unavailable to people of this culture
DAVID & GOLIATH	Answer to major question (e.g., cancer) has been found by "little man" where the might of national or industrial bodies have failed
JUSTICE	Cure is available to those whose attitudes and beliefs mark them as worthy of it

All of these factors—the personal attributes of the complementary medicine practitioners and the philosophical aspects of the remedy itself—offer the patients a more supportive feeling in the consultation, an expectation of being more involved in their own care, and of greater hope.

So now, let's address the issue of greater hope in some detail.

Research has shown that one of the top three reasons why people go to complementary medicine practitioners is that they believe the remedies work—and that offers them hope.

Some—perhaps a lot—of that hope comes from stories of unexpected or miraculous responses, and often of cures. I feel very strongly that it is important to view stories such as these with some sense of perspective, and I am going to discuss some alternative explanations for some of them in the next section.

I must stress the fact that I am not being curmudgeonly and purely negative about these stories. I think this is important because in the two and one-half years that I spent investigating such stories, I saw that reports of apparently inexplicable miracles had a very wide circulation, and were responsible for much of the attraction and pull of complementary medicine.

In all of the stories that I investigated, I found everyday explanations that had not been considered, and I think it is important to be aware of these more mundane explanations in order to avoid having hopes falsely raised and then suffering deep disappointment.

Possible Explanations of Apparently Inexplicable Miracles

During the making of the television series *Magic or Medicine?*, I spent two and a half years investigating dozens of stories of miraculous cures. We had invited people to write to us if they had a story of a miraculous or an unexpected benefit, and we investigated all the letters we received.

In every single case, there was a mundane and everyday explanation for that benefit. I think it's worth listing those types of explanations, because, as I said, these stories are often a major reason why people think that there is something new and revolutionary about a treatment.

In the cases I investigated, these were the main types of alternative everyday explanations:

No Facts

Some stories are passed from person to person, and acquire more authority, credibility, and details with each retelling. For this reason, it can be very difficult to get to the bottom of a story that at first appears to be totally credible.

For example, I spoke to a woman in her mid-fifties who had telephoned our researcher to say that she had been cured of bowel cancer by herbal treatments recommended to her by an *iridologist* seven years earlier. (An iridologist is a complementary medicine practitioner who diagnoses disease by looking at the iris of the eye.)

She told the researcher that she had previously been seen at a local hospital by a conventional gastroenterologist who had done a biopsy and told her that she had bowel cancer and that she needed surgery. She had refused the surgery, had gone to the iridologist, and had been taking the herbal remedy for many years. She was alive and well—clearly showing, she said, that this herbal remedy could indeed cure bowel cancer.

The researcher was very impressed by the story which, if it were true, would have been enormously important. So I asked the researcher to obtain the exact date of the biopsy so that I could have it reevaluated. I suspected that the biopsy would not show an invasive cancer, but would show a kind of polyp that was premalignant. In other words I thought that the patient probably had had, not a cancer, but a polyp that had a *chance* of becoming a cancer.

The woman told our researcher the exact date and location of the biopsy, so I contacted the pathology department of that hospital. We searched the pathology records using three different spellings of the woman's name and several variations on her birth date. We also searched records for the previous two years and the two subsequent years. There was no record of any biopsy.

At this point I telephoned the woman myself. (I had not spoken to her directly before that.) She confirmed what she had said to the researcher. When I asked her about the biopsy, she then said she had *not* had a biopsy, but that the gastroenterologist had told her that he did not like the look of her colon. In other words, there was no actual proof that this particular patient had ever had cancer, or even a risk of it.

Now, I am not saying that this woman deliberately misled our researcher, but I do feel that she gave in to wishful thinking. She very much appreciated the attention of her iridologist and was, in her view, simply trying to amplify the benefit of what she thought the iridologist had done for her.

Of course, the story was immensely powerful and entirely credible. Three other members of our office staff who heard this story firmly believed, when they first heard it, that it was proof that cancer could be cured by herbal remedies. It just happened not to be true. And it was only because I happened to be in a position to check the crucial evidence, that it was possible to see there was none.

If I been unable to search the records of that hospital, this story would have gone unchallenged, and might have been accepted as clear proof that a complementary medicine treatment had cured bowel cancer.

There are many stories like that.

You often hear of a person who is at "four removes" who has been miraculously cured of, say, lung cancer. (I call stories like this "anecdotes of the hairdresser's daughter's friend's grandmother." Four degrees of separation between you and the protagonist.) When you chase up the facts, you find out that it wasn't lung cancer, it was an attack of bronchitis, and her doctor was trying to persuade her to give up smoking. But the original story has already gained wide circulation and great credibility.

It is very difficult for a person who has been diagnosed with a cancer to think calmly and objectively about stories like this. They may feel impolite or even insensitive and churlish to ask where the story came from, or to ask if there really was evidence of the cancer. (Probably every re-teller of the story would claim that a biopsy had been done anyway.)

All I can suggest is that when you hear about a miraculous cure you remember that one possible explanation is that "the facts aren't there." Keeping that sense of perspective—almost skepticism—might help you not to get sucked in and so not have your hopes falsely raised.

Premature Reporting

Another reason why anecdotes of individual cases may be misleading is that results are often reported prematurely. A patient may sincerely believe that he or she is cured by a remedy and that an unexpected or miraculous remission has occurred, and may say so. But it may be too early to make that statement.

This kind of premature pronouncement will of course do no harm to the patient. After all, it may be beneficial to believe that you are doing well and to have a genuinely positive attitude. However, the story may mislead other people into believing that the treatment has a genuine effect when it does not. The most famous example of this was the story of the much-loved movie actor Steve McQueen.

McQueen had a mesothelioma, a rare and extremely aggressive cancer which in his case occurred in the abdomen. His conventional physicians told him that there was nothing further they could do, so he went to a private clinic in Mexico. There he was given a variety of treatments including herbal remedies, colonic irrigation, diet supplements, and meditation.

He was so impressed by the way he felt that he made a public broadcast on Mexican radio thanking the president and people of Mexico for allowing the clinic to exist and allowing him to be cured of his disease. On the recording, he sounded extremely ill, and in fact he died a few weeks later, after a hazardous part of his treatment at the clinic that involved surgery.

The point is that at the time that radio broadcast went out, listeners all over the world believed that he had been cured. In some places it was announced on the news that he had been cured. And McQueen was so loved and adored, that large numbers of people believed it. (In fact, there is a tiny group of people who *still* believe that he was cured, and that he was murdered on the orders of conventional physicians who did not want their method of treatment to be challenged by this Mexican clinic.)

So, a story like that raises hopes falsely. Because it tells us what we would like to hear, it is very difficult to be cautious in greeting the news.

If an icon such as McQueen says, "I have been cured," it is very difficult for anyone to reply or even think, "Perhaps things are going well now, but to call it a cure may be overoptimistic."

All I am saying is that you may need time (not just facts) before you can truly judge the worth of a story. It is always difficult to stop and wait, when you want so badly to believe what you are being told and you hope so strongly that it is true.

Variations in Natural History
Another possible explanation for apparently miraculous cures is the variability of many forms of cancer. Cancers do not always behave in a uniform way.

Imagine a particularly aggressive form of cancer that, let us say, usually results in the patient's death within two years in 95 percent of cases. That still means that one out of every twenty patients will be alive beyond that time—that is not miraculous or unusual, it is simply the way things happen in a small percentage of cases

Over the years, I have seen many cases where a matter of statistics seemed to be miraculous. One of the first patients I looked after as a resident was a man with acute myeloid leukemia. At that time, there was virtually no treatment for it, and yet this young man was alive and completely well nearly three years after diagnosis.

He was an immensely likable man, and we were all very glad for him, but the disease did eventually progress. Similarly, I remember a woman in her early sixties with malignant melanoma that had spread to her liver (many years after the initial diagnosis). She remained alive and functioning for over four years with those metastases in the liver— something which happens very rarely.

Another patient of mine at present has breast cancer with secondaries in the lungs which have remained basically the same size for over three years, despite the fact that she refuses to take any treatment. These are all examples of how impressive and memorable individual stories can be if they concern something that is very different from the average course of events.

Simultaneous Conventional Therapy

An even more important explanation is the possibility that a patient may be taking conventional medicine at the same time as complementary medicine—and may not even realize it.

For example, a few years ago I interviewed a woman who was a cofounder of a very well-known complementary cancer help center in Britain. She herself had had breast cancer and had written about it in a book which detailed the various complementary remedies that she had used. At one point, her breast cancer recurred on the chest wall and her oncologist recommended that she take tamoxifen. She wrote that she thought about it for a time and decided not to. She went on to write about various herbs and other treatments that she took, and then said that her conventional doctor was very surprised to find, a few months later, that the cancer was shrinking.

When I interviewed her, I asked her directly why, in those circumstances, she had decided not to take tamoxifen. She replied that, in fact, she had been taking tamoxifen for several years during this whole period.

In the way she said it, it was clear that she did not realize that tamoxifen is a conventional anticancer hormone agent and causes regression of breast cancer (if it is receptor-positive, as hers was) in nearly 60 percent of cases.

In other words, the course of her disease was exactly what we would have expected in a case of recurrent estrogen-receptor positive breast cancer being treated with conventional tamoxifen.

Another woman, whom I interviewed in Mexico, told me point blank that she was not taking any medication for her cancer (breast cancer with positive lymph nodes) except the complementary medicine remedies given to her by the Tijuana clinic.

After our filmed interview, I asked her again, and it was only at this stage that she remembered that she had indeed been taking tamoxifen (she only knew it by its brand name, hence the confusion) every day since her surgery two years ago. Had we shown the filmed interview as she gave it, the viewer would have believed that the complementary medicine remedies alone were controlling her breast cancer.

So these examples illustrate another type of explanation for an apparent miracle. It is important to realize the difficulty in judging any statement about the efficacy of a complementary medicine remedy (as opposed to a conventional treatment). These claims need to be evaluated carefully, because many patients receive, knowingly or unknowingly, conventional treatment at the same time.

Misinterpretation

Apart from these rather black or white factual issues, there are several ways in which it is possible to misinterpret what a doctor says, and this may lead to an outcome that is, apparently, miraculous or unexpected.

One is selective recall. Discussing the prognosis is one of the most emotionally charged conversations imaginable. As a result, what a patient remembers and recounts may not necessarily be what the doctor said.

A lot of people will ask their doctor directly, "How long have I got?" Many doctors, myself included, feel that we have to give an honest answer, that we are not allowed to avoid the discussion altogether. Because no one can predict exactly what is going to happen, however, it is usually possible to give only the most likely range of possibilities. So that is what we do.

For example there might be a type of cancer in which, in an advanced stage, 50 percent of the patients will be alive at two years, and 5 percent will be alive at five years. It would be fair to say that the prognosis probably is measured in a small number of years for most people, but a few will do better than that—and I have said that to many patients.

The patient may then ask me whether that means that the prognosis could be less than a year, say six months or less. Since a few people in this situation will die of the disease in a short time—say less than six months—I would usually say, "Yes, that could happen but it is not very likely."

The patient might then ask, "So, do you mean that I might not be around in three months?"

I would probably reply, "Well, that is not very likely, but it could happen."

The patient might then go home, where a spouse or a relative will certainly ask what the doctor said, and the patient might well reply, "The doctor gave me three months."

If this patient then uses a complementary medicine remedy and is alive at two years—as half of all such patients would be anyway—often the credit for that apparent extension of the prognosis is given to the complementary remedy, which might then be credited with producing miraculous remissions in patients with this type of cancer.

A second source of confusion is misunderstanding. Sometimes, with all the stress and worry surrounding a hospital visit, it is easy to misinterpret and misremember what the medical team said, occasionally leading to a totally different interpretation of what is happening.

During the making of our television series, I received a letter from a man who said that three years previously he had had a sarcoma on his left thigh. He wrote that CT scans of his lungs had shown metastases, which would usually mean that his chance of surviving would be very small.

His doctors had treated the tumor on his thigh (with surgery and radiotherapy to the leg) but had given him no treatment for the metastases. He had then embarked on a major lifestyle change. He took up intensive prayer, meditation, psychotherapy, dietary change and exercise, and now, three years later, he was completely well.

Once again, several members of the production staff took this as clear evidence that lifestyle change including prayer and meditation could, of itself, control the growth of cancer.

We visited the hospitals where he had been treated and had had the lung CT scans. In fact, his first CT scan had shown two small shadows at the bottom of the left lung which his doctors thought *might* be metastases but could be other things, including little pieces of scar tissue. They had told him exactly that. They also said that they would repeat the scans every three months. If the shadows got bigger, that would prove they were metastases: if they stayed the same, that would suggest they were scars.

In fact, the shadows stayed the same size for more than three years, which meant that they were scars after all. I later found out that the man had had some exposure to asbestos when he was younger, asbestos being one of the substances that often leaves tiny little scars in the lungs.

When we later interviewed the patient, he said that he did remember being told that the shadows had remained the same size and therefore were not secondaries. However, with our production team as evidence, it was easy for observers to accept this patient's version of events at face value, and therefore to believe that lifestyle changes could control cancer.

Wrong Diagnosis

In some cases, the diagnosis is wrong. This is not very common, but it does happen, particularly with certain cancers where distinguishing a true cancer from a nonmalignant condition may be difficult. For example, occasionally a small-cell lung cancer might be indistinguishable from bronchial-adenoma, a benign condition.

A patient of mine, who is very much alive and well, had breast cancer diagnosed fourteen years ago. That in itself is not remarkable: many patients may be cured after primary surgery. Nine years ago she developed a lymph node in the neck and a biopsy was done which showed recurrent cancer. Recurrence in the neck is not curable.

At that time, standard treatment was to remove the ovaries, which changes the hormonal environment and often causes breast cancers to shrink, as this neck lump did. However, shortly afterwards, she developed another lump in the neck which was monitored for several years and which did not change in size.

Her doctors believed that she now had a second recurrence of her breast cancer, which was, for some unknown reason, stable. At that point she moved and was referred her to me because I was geographically the nearest.

With the benefit of not having her assessed before, I was puzzled by the lump in her neck and ordered a CT scan. The lump turned out to be, not cancer, but a malformation of the vertebral body, called a *cervical rib*.

Having had biopsy-proven cancer in the neck nearly ten years previously, this woman had (probably) been cured by the removal of her ovaries and now was free of cancer, although she had a cervical rib. Had she been taking any complementary medicine remedies, her case might have been widely publicized as a case of incurable cancer that was held in check for a decade by the remedy. As it was, she had probably been cured (although such cases are very unusual) by the second operation.

Spontaneous Remissions

In a very few cases, a cancer may disappear completely without any treatment whatsoever.

This is called *spontaneous remission* and it's a rare event. In fact one pathologist, William Boyd, documented in great detail a large number of such instances in a book he published in 1961. He estimated that approximately one in every 100,000 cases of cancer will show spontaneous remission. In his documentation, collected from data extending over a hundred years, more than half of the proven cases of spontaneous remission came from four types of tumor. Those types were: renal-cell cancer, melanoma (the pigmented cancer of the skin), neuroblastoma (a rare cancer of childhood) and choriocarcinoma (also a rare cancer of the placenta). In the other half of the cases, there were one or two examples of spontaneous remission in almost every type of cancer.

These facts are very important. First, they prove that almost any type of cancer can remit without apparent cause. Second, they show that spontaneous remission is much more common among those four rare types of cancer than it is among all the others.

Feeling Better vs. Getting Better

But the most common, and by far the most important, explanation of the unexpected benefit is the important fact that there is a difference between getting better and feeling better.

Most patients (in fact, I think it's virtually 100 percent) who try complementary medicine come out of the experience *feeling* better—whether or not they are *getting* better.

Furthermore, they may feel better even while tests (say, blood tests of liver function or measurements of the tumor or of the arm) show that the cancer is progressing. As one patient said, "Feeling good is good in itself." Feelings of improvement are an end in themselves, even though they should not be confused with a true regression of the cancer.

Sometimes there are additional reasons why the patient may feel better.

At a faith-healing demonstration in Britain, recorded for television, a healer brought on a nine-year-old girl who had a rare cancer in the bones. (It was, I later found out, a neuroblastoma.) She was on very high doses of morphine and could walk only with difficulty. In the presence of over ten thousand people, the healer encouraged her to get out of her wheelchair, which she did. She walked across the stage and the healer told her (on television) that the next time she saw her doctor, she would be told that she had no cancer in her bones.

Sadly, he was wrong and the girl died a few weeks later. Why had she been able to walk? Partially because the healer and the entire audience so wanted her to get well, that she overcame (probably subconsciously) her feelings of pain and was able for a moment to stand and walk.

A few months after this, I experienced the value of that kind of support for myself. I went to a healing ceremony in Mexico at which, each year, it is thought that a charismatic healer called *El Niño* is reincarnated inside the body of one of his followers. I was there to observe the ceremony. But (without my knowledge) the film producer told the healer that I was ill and partially crippled (both of which are quite true).

Suddenly, in the middle of the ceremony, the healer turned to me, and the audience also focused on me. Without warning I was suddenly in the center of over a hundred people's gaze, and wishes and prayers for my recovery.

Although I did not believe in the reincarnation or the healing powers of *El Niño*, the feeling that I experienced in that instant was tremendous. It was like being warmed and wrapped up in a cozy blanket of affection and regard. I felt—as I have never felt at any other time—that here were scores of people sincerely wanting me to get well. It was a truly remarkable and pleasant moment. It did not make any difference to my physical disability, but it certainly made me feel wonderful. And it taught me the value of other people wanting you to get well.

In my own experience I have not yet seen a miracle cure or remission with complementary medicine that cannot be explained in a straightforward everyday way.

To me, that means that stories of apparent miracle cures should be judged with a small measure of skepticism. If it sounds too good to be true, it probably is!

But stories like the ones above travel wide and they travel fast, and they raise every listener's hopes. If they later turn out not to be factual, which is what has happened with all of them so far, then it is the patient with a cancer diagnosis who suffers the harm, and experiences the disappointment and dismay.

"Can't I Try Complementary Medicines Anyway?"

The short answer is, in my opinion, "Sure."

I genuinely do not mind my patients trying any complementary remedy that they wish, *as long as they have realistic expectations of it*, and will not be crushed with disappointment if it doesn't do them any physical good.

Now this is my opinion. Some oncologists are more rigid and often object to their patients taking complementary medicines—partly because of the rare possibility of interactions between the complementary and the conventional medicines. I consider it much more important for patients to make sure they think about *why* they are trying the remedy, and what hopes or expectations they have.

So, to summarize my own view, I am asking you to accept that any remedy touted as effective against cancer may not be, but even so, with the right attitude, you may still want to try it. When it comes to deciding whether you should still go to Mexico or Switzerland or Zaire or Berlin or try that herbal remedy or the ozone therapy or the laetrile or the shark cartilage, I personally believe that it matters more *why* you do something than *whether* you do it or not.

If you try a complementary medicine remedy with the attitude that it would be nice it worked and would not be a disaster if it didn't, and if you can afford the money and the time, then you will lose nothing. And you may feel a fair bit better in yourself for doing it.

If, on the other hand, you feel desperate, you want more than anything else to be cured, and you are prepared to sell anything and go anywhere to get a cure, then you are setting yourself up for serious disappointment. And you may later find that you have lost both time and money, when both are scarce.

So, in some respects the most important question is not, "Shall I go?" Rather, it is, "What are my feelings about going, and what am I expecting?"

It is really difficult to keep a cool head when you are a patient with cancer, and you feel that your clock is ticking, and your conventional doctors have told you the situation is not curable.

Yet I hope that the information in this section will at least give a sense of perspective and perhaps allow you a bit of intellectual breathing space, both to evaluate what you are being told (by anyone) and to decide what it is that you really want to do.

"How Do I
Get Back on Track?"

Living Your Life

The word *cancer* rings all the alarm bells and makes it almost impossible to carry on with life in a normal way.

The sense of emergency often pushes everybody—patient and family alike—into an emergency mode that affects almost every aspect of daily life, including the most basic things such as the simple activity of talking to other people.

You need to get back to your normal habits and patterns—to restore the situation as far as possible to the way it was. And that is not always easy. This section will give you some general guidelines that will help you live well—not merely survive—after the diagnosis turns everything topsy-turvy.

The diagnosis of a cancer creates many far reaching ripples of stress and emotion which spread out through your whole family and circle of friends. So, I also set out some simple and practical tips which may help you to restore your normal patterns of living.

I will start with how we use some important words, which subtly affect the way you think about getting back on track.

Living Well?

There is a problem with the word *survivor*, particularly when it is used in *cancer survivor*. It implies that almost everybody else has died.

This might seem to be a trivial shade of meaning, or even a form of political correctness. But in my view it isn't.

Let me give you an example from outside the world of medicine. In July 2005, an Airbus plane crashed and burst into flames shortly after landing at Toronto airport. Every single one of the 309 passengers and crew got out alive and there were no major or life-threatening injuries. The media coverage consistently employed the word *survivor*, and also the word *miracle*, both of which were totally justifiable.

The point is that when a plane crashes on landing, there are almost always a large number of deaths, and this expectation is reflected in the use of the word *survivor*. All 309 people who clambered out of the wreckage are genuine survivors because in similar situations many people die.

But a diagnosis of cancer is not a plane crash. And although some cancers carry a high mortality rate, many do not. As I have pointed out repeatedly in this book, to lump them all together and call anyone who is alive a *cancer survivor* maintains the idea that most people with a cancer diagnosis are expected to die.

Many times in recent years well-known personalities and celebrities have been called *breast cancer survivors*. Several of them, we later found out, had small breast tumors which had not spread to the lymph nodes—situations in which the chance of the cancer not coming back is around 95 percent. It is absolutely wonderful that these particular individuals are alive and are talking about their experiences (which would never have been publicized a decade ago). But to call them *survivors* gives the impression that all but a few breast cancer patients will die.

The discussion is right—but the word is, slightly, wrong.

Surviving versus Thriving

The word *surviving* also implies that the main focus of the person's life is simply the fact that she or he is alive. Surviving means *not dying*, and doesn't imply any more than that.

We have another word, *thriving*, which implies a lot more. To thrive means to do well, and it implies a good quality of life. It's a neat word— but there's no such word as *thrivership*. Perhaps there ought to be, and perhaps there will be soon, but at the moment we can't talk about the art of thrivership, or thrivership programs, or anything like that.

So we need a new word or phrase, and the one that seems most suitable to me is the phrase *living well*.

It seems to carry all the right meanings and implications. If a person says, "I had colon cancer seven years ago and I'm living well," it says everything.

So, just for the moment, perhaps we can all make a conscious effort to replace *survivor* with *living well*. It's a couple of extra words, but it opens a totally different range of meaning.

Now we can look at the elements of living well—and how to do it.

First Things First: Some General Guidelines

Here are a few simple guidelines that my patients have told me about. They work in practice and are fairly easy to remember.

DON'T SET THE BAR TOO HIGH—SET REALISTIC TARGETS. We all have a tendency to reach too high. In the recovery phase after the initial diagnosis and (usually) surgery, it may be tempting to want to get right back up on your feet. The problem is, if that doesn't happen, you will be very disappointed and daunted. And that disappointment will probably prolong your recovery.

So, even if you have always been the kind of person that could do in one hour what took everyone else three hours, go easy on yourself and don't expect too much of yourself in the first few weeks. Even in a healthy person a general anesthetic often produces fatigue and loss of energy for at least a couple of weeks. So don't set the bar too high.

DON'T GO BACK TO WORK TOO EARLY. After surgery especially, but also if you are working at the time of diagnosis, resist the temptation to rush back to work as soon as possible.

A lot of people have a tendency to define themselves (and their worth) in terms of their work. If they are doing well at work, they feel they are worthwhile people, if not, they may feel a bit worthless. If that is the case with you, be aware that you can tarnish your good reputation if you go back to work while you are still feeling unwell and turn in a substandard performance. Unfortunately the memory of that lingers. You lose points and, sadly, support and sympathy as well.

ACKNOWLEDGE YOUR BAD DAYS. There will be many good days when you feel optimistic that you can handle anything. But there will also be some bad days when you think that things will never improve, and you feel daunted and oppressed. On those days, you might well feel that you don't have the energy to change anything and you never will.

Here's a useful tip: if you're having a bad day, acknowledge it to yourself. *Tell yourself* that you are having a bad day. Accept it, find something else to occupy your attention, and start over again, later or on the next day.

It's not just you. It's a universal phenomenon. We all have some bad days and some good days. Pretending to yourself that a bad day is actually a good day can make you feel even worse: it usually adds guilt, and a sense of inadequacy, a suspicion that you ought not to be having down times.

TAKE SEVERAL SMALL STEPS INSTEAD OF A FEW BIG ONES. That's the secret of instilling a bit of confidence. And one thing that helps most people is visible achievement.

There may be days when you can physically manage only to climb one flight of stairs, or psychologically you can manage to read only the front page of the newspaper. If that is the case, take those small steps and quit while you're ahead.

When you're recovering from an illness, the scale of your achievements suddenly narrows, and your horizons may not extend further than the one flight of stairs or the front page of the newspaper. If that is so, acknowledge that to yourself.

It is not the way you'd like it to be, but it's the way it is.

GIVE YOURSELF MORE TIME THAN USUAL. Part of the difference between a chore and a pleasure is time. Even an activity that is pleasurable can become unpleasant if you have to rush through it and there is no time to enjoy it. By the same token, even something you don't like doing can become moderately enjoyable if you have enough time set aside for it.

That works well if you're healthy, and even better if you're not.

YOU CAN PLAN FOR THE WORST AND HOPE FOR THE BEST AT THE SAME TIME. These two activities don't cancel each other out. (Have a look at what I say about the many effects and aspects of hope on pages 211–217.)

Never be afraid to plan for bad outcomes. Those plans are not self-fulfilling prophesies. In fact the opposite is true: once you have decided how you would respond if bad things happen, you can actually stop thinking about them. And you will find that you can actually concentrate more—not less—on your day-to-day living.

Support: *"What Is It and What Does It Feel Like?"*

We all know roughly what we mean by the words *support* or *supportive*, but when we think about it carefully, it's actually quite difficult to define the main ingredients.

Together with Dr. Walter Baile, who is head of psychiatry at the M.D. Anderson Cancer Center, University of Texas, I have described *support* as consisting of two essential components: acknowledging the way the other person is feeling (see the empathic response, pages 182–183) and advocacy, meaning the act of taking steps to try to resolve the unmet needs of the patient:

Support = Acknowledgement + Advocacy

In other words, to give support you have to do (at the very least) two things. First, you have to identify what the other person is feeling, either by actions or demeanor or by words, and show that you acknowledge it and the events or circumstances that triggered it. Second, you have to understand and acknowledge a person's "shopping list" of wishes or needs and take steps to find where these can be met, as far as possible. To be supportive, you have to try to find a solution or information, even if it is not possible to give the patient what he or she ultimately wants (e.g., cure of the tumor).

Support is a much more a matter of *process*—the way you do something or attempt to do it—than it is of *outcome*—the results that you achieve or fail to achieve.

Talking with Other People: *"It Ain't What You Say, It's the Way You Say It"*

Although we do it all the time, talking with other people is something we rarely focus on or consciously think about.

Hence, most people do not realize that you can use *strategies* for communication: ways of approaching difficult topics. You can, in other words, consciously decide on an approach to communication.

In this section I will show you how to do that. I should add that I have been teaching strategies for communication and communication skills for the last twenty years to physicians and medical students all over the world. Quite a lot of what you will read in this section has now been tested in research studies. It works—as you'll see for yourself!

"What Good Does Talking Do?"

As we all know (but never properly admit to ourselves) human contact—communication during which one person changes the way another person feels and/or thinks—is exceptionally important.

A change in the way we feel dramatically alters our ability to cope.

One of the most dreaded aspects of any illness (and this has been documented for many years) is the sensation of being alone and isolated. If you feel cut off from the people around you, you will be prone to depression and many other symptoms of withdrawal and "shutting down."

Communication with those around you changes all this. Which is why this whole subject is so important.

Furthermore, your communication skills and abilities say something about you—whether you mean them to or not. Many years ago, doctors were not accustomed to having open and honest communication with their patients. And even if they wanted to do it, they had no idea which techniques would work and which would not. As a result, many doctors were perceived as being cold, insensitive, and uncaring. I have spoken to several doctors who were thought to be cold and insensitive and found that they were no such thing. They simply had no idea how to respond or what to say, so they said nothing, which was interpreted as sullenness and lack of warmth. Once they were shown a few relatively simple communication techniques, the impression that they gave to their patients improved dramatically.

The same is true for you.

Whether you are the patient (by which I mean the person with a cancer diagnosis) or a friend, the way in which you communicate—and particularly the way you listen and how you respond—will visibly change the relationship between the two of you and alter the outcome of the discussions you have.

Furthermore, as you discuss something you are worried about or unsure of, you may realize, as you talk, that you have begun to solve the problem. The way you phrase the question often tells you the answer.

In other words, good communication not only establishes genuine contact between you, but also helps resolve issues and puts unresolved questions into perspective.

I'll start here with some tips for the patient when talking with family and friends and with the medical team, then I'll continue with a section for friends and family members, giving them some tips for talking with and listening to the patient.

Now, there are no secrets here: anyone can read any of these sections. I've written the sections separately only because each party is starting from a different place, and may have problems which are quite specific to that particular position.

Talking with Friends and Family (Tips for The Person with a Cancer Diagnosis)

In an ideal world, people with medical conditions would not have to come up with a strategy for talking about that condition with their friends and family. It would be natural and intuitive.

Unfortunately, the word *cancer* is so emotionally loaded and so fraught with overtones of gloom and dread that it often makes ordinary normal communication impossible.

Therefore, you do have to have some strategies for how you can approach the subject of your diagnosis or condition with your friends.

It isn't fair: in theory, you shouldn't have to plan how you discuss your situation. It *should* be easy and spontaneous. In our present society, however, this type of conversation *isn't* easy, and so you do need ways to make it easier.

The Cauldron of Emotions

One of my patients described her feelings after her diagnosis as a boiling cauldron of emotions. That cauldron contained all kinds of emotions and thoughts bubbling and boiling together. Some of them were hers and some of them came from our society's reactions and attitudes to the word *cancer*.

I think it is worth spending a moment or two analyzing what that patient said, because she is absolutely right. If you have just been told that you have one of the two hundred types of cancer, you will experience a complex mixture of emotions, fears, and thoughts. Some of those will be very specific to you and will have been formed by your own previous experiences and reactions to adverse events. Some of them will be preformed by our society. In other words, some of the discomfort you feel comes from your own experience and some of it comes from the attitudes of other people.

Let's deal with those separately.

Your feelings

You may experience any or many of the following feelings, and it may be helpful for you to know that other people, in similar situations, experience them too. Which means that we can correctly call them *normal*.

SHOCK: We all know what shock is: a major and unpleasant surprise. No matter how prepared you are, the diagnosis of a cancer is almost always a shock. Even if your particular cancer has already been cured by the time the biopsy has been done, for many people the word *cancer* in any context, at any time, immediately provokes an automatic reaction of shock.

DISBELIEF: Disbelief is such a common feeling it would be fair to call it almost universal. Everyone tends to experience a sense of unreality, a feeling of "this can't be happening to me," when they first hear a cancer diagnosis. The important point to hold on to is that this reaction is usual. It's not your fault and it's not cowardice or stupidity that causes this reaction.

DENIAL: For quite a lot of people that feeling of disbelief is accompanied by a desire to shut out the news, to deny it. There is a lot written and broadcast about denial and some of it seems to suggest that denial is somehow always harmful and should be immediately confronted and broken down.

In my view, and in the view of many other professionals experienced in this area, that is simply not true. Many people use denial as a perfectly normal and valuable method of dealing with threatening or overwhelming news *when they first hear it.* In other words, denial is a normal human coping strategy which allows you to take serious news on board without having it totally swamp you. It is only when denial is prolonged, going on for many weeks or months, and causes breakdown in communications between the patient and family or healthcare team that it becomes a problem. So if you come to realize that you are using denial, or if someone close to you points that out, you do not need to chastise yourself or feel that you must hurry to overcome it. It may well be a normal reaction which in time—a few days perhaps, or a couple of weeks—will allow you to accept the news and deal constructively with it.

AWKWARDNESS: Apart from shock, disbelief, and denial—all of which make it difficult for you to talk about your situation—another problem is that you may not be *accustomed* to talking about deeply personal and intimate matters. In fact, many people aren't. In a lot of families and friendships, deeply intimate concerns are not talked about. Or if they are, they're not talked about easily and supportively. If that has been your pattern in the past, then of course you are going to find it difficult if you want (or need) to talk about your feelings at this moment of crisis. Again, being aware of this will help.

FEAR: As I've said so many times, the word *cancer* itself brings with it so many associations of dread and fear and inevitable gloom, that a rush of fear is also almost universal.

PANIC: I think that panic is basically the same thing as fear, but at a higher level of intensity. When fear reaches a certain level, it affects our ability to think clearly and make rational decisions. I think that is what we all understand by the word *panic*. It is fear at a level high enough to overwhelm our decision-making processes.

ANGER: Most people feel some degree of anger at their body for letting them down, for throwing an unexpected and large obstacle into their path and interfering with their plans. This anger is often mixed with, and perhaps partly caused by, disappointment and a feeling that, "The body has failed me and that means I'm a failure too." Again, these are feelings that most people have: they are not true or untrue, not appropriate or inappropriate, they are simply what most people experience to some degree.

GUILT: Guilt is also very common, but guilt is almost a taboo subject and is rarely talked about. Guilt is the emotional component of self-blame.

If you feel a sense of guilt, it means that you are attributing a measure of blame to yourself for your condition, whether that is appropriate or not. In fact you are more likely to experience guilt if the condition is entirely random and you have made no contribution to its cause.

FRUSTRATION AND LOSS OF CONTROL: We are living in a society in which people expect more and more control over the many aspects of their daily lives. We expect to be able to watch the television programs we want, to buy the foods we want, and to get to work in a specified amount of time. We also expect to get frustrated if something goes wrong and these things do not happen.

DESPAIR: This emotion is associated with the perception, even if it is totally false, that there is no hope. One of the most common triggers for a reaction of despair is simply not knowing what the options for treatment are, and what the future prospects are likely to be. As one patient put it, "If you don't know what can be done, you immediately jump to the conclusion that nothing can be done."

Despair is a common and normal reaction, and one of the most direct and immediate ways to counteract it is to learn and understand more about the cancer and the way it can be treated. (That's why I wrote this book in the first place, to help you with that.)

HUMOR: A lot of people use humor to help them through bad times. Sometimes there is a feeling lurking in the background that this is somehow wrong, that some things should never be joked about. I believe that humor is a useful adaptive response and is a coping strategy. If you use a little of it to help you cope, the end result is the only thing that matters.

Without getting too grandiose, we can define humor as a deliberate and knowing diversion or side-road away from an expected response or sequence of events. Because this activity, departing from what is expected, is a deliberate and conscious choice, humor can be not only good for the person who initiates it, but also good for the communal feeling between that person and the people who hear it. By sharing in the humor they reinforce their sense of contact with each other. In other words, humor is a very good bonding material if it is used *after* taking the serious issues seriously.

So if you are the kind of person who usually uses a touch of humor when the going gets rough, then don't feel worried about doing that now. Humor allows you to gets things into some sort of perspective, it allows you to draw a frame around the threat, and (usually) it allows other people to relax a bit while they are with you.

Society's Attitudes to Serious Illness

Above we listed a few of the emotions and responses to a cancer diagnosis that arise from inside you. There are also emotions and attitudes that are pre-set by society. In the same way that a society decides how it is going to react to words such as *terrorist* or *pandemic*, to some degree some of the connotations attached to the word *cancer* are pre-fabricated by the society we live in.

At the moment our society tends to value highly the qualities of youth, wealth, and health. This is not necessarily wrong, or morally lax. But it does mean that anyone who is old, poor, or sick tends to get marginalized. In any community that esteems the young and the fit, people will feel downgraded and pushed aside as they become older or sicker, especially if either of those is accompanied by a decrease in wealth.

So some of the many feelings in your cauldron may be partly a reflection of society's attitude to illness in general, and there are several elements to this.

THE STIGMA OF BAD LUCK: We tend to value success and the people who succeed. Society may acknowledge that luck plays a part in that success, but that is generally lip service, and the people who do well usually attribute their success to their own efforts and worthy qualities.

If a person experiences bad luck, then, he or she often finds there is a stigma that goes along with it. Society tends to shun people who are having bad luck, as if the bad luck itself were contagious. Hence, if you are experiencing an illness that society regards as potentially serious, you may find that some of your more superficial contacts fade or disappear.

SHAME: With the loss of social esteem and status comes (occasionally) a sense of shame—it is almost as if anyone who has any form of cancer is somehow a lesser individual. Not a pariah or a leper, but somehow lower in the pecking order. This is common when the diagnosis is a cancer, but not when the diagnosis is emphysema, for example.

ROLE REDEFINITION: The same root causes are responsible for the uneasy way in which you have to adjust to a new definition of your role, even if it is only temporary.

If you are a wage-earner or contribute in other ways to your family life or to your community, it is extremely upsetting not to be able to fill that role.

The emotions above are just some of the many ingredients that may be bubbling alongside each other in the emotional cauldron. These feelings are not instantly fixable, not like a noise in your car that can be fixed once you get to the mechanic. Feelings like these need a bit of *thinking about* and a fair amount of *talking about*—which is why talking to your friends is so important.

No matter how you are feeling or what you are feeling, at some point things are likely to be easier if you can find someone with whom you can talk.

"Who Should I Talk To?"

Again, in an ideal world, each of us would have a confiding and close relationship (perhaps with our spouse or partner) as well as a wide circle of supportive friends with whom we could discuss our innermost feelings.

That is the ideal, and a few lucky people do have that. Most of us, however, have something less perfect. And some of us seem (at first) to have no one we can talk to.

So the first question is this: if you want to talk, who is the best person to talk to?

Well, who do you *usually* talk to about big problems? Who was the first person you wanted to go to when something big went wrong in the past? If there is someone to whom you've always confided your serious worries or problems, then of course that person should be at the top of your list now.

If you do not have a close confidant, ask yourself who you could imagine talking to, who would make you feel most comfortable when discussing difficult problems.

It might be anyone. There's no universal "best person." It may be your spouse, your closest friend, your mother, sister, brother, priest, or it may even be somebody you quite like but haven't (until now) been on close terms with. In fact, sometimes people with cancer find it rather daunting or intimidating to talk to close family about it. Sometimes they actually find it easier to speak to someone relatively distant, such as a business partner, first.

If you simply have no idea whom to talk to, discuss that with your doctor or nurse or someone else on your medical team. Also, try to find out more about the support groups in your area or associated with your cancer center. (You can also visit the Web sites mentioned at the end of this book.)

"How Do I Ask for What I Want?"

Once you've identified the person with whom you stand the best chance of having supportive conversation, what next? Here are a few hints that may make that conversation easier:

TRY TO DECIDE WHICH THINGS ARE REALLY IMPORTANT: It's a bit like making an agenda in your mind. If you leave the more important things till the end, you'll tend to be preoccupied and edgy while you're talking about the other stuff. Quite often there are only two or three things that are right at the top of the list. So decide what they are and go for them first.

TRY TO GIVE A HEADLINE OR SIGNPOST FIRST: Giving a headline or "signposting" what you are going to talk about is fairly common in business transactions, but we don't often do it in normal social conversation. However, these are not normal social circumstances, so you are allowed to do things in a slightly different way.

You can begin by saying, "Look, I want to say a couple of things that are on my mind. Is that OK with you?" or "There's something that's really worrying me. Can we talk for a minute?"

This alerts the other person to the fact that what follows is something that really matters. They will almost certainly switch on fully and focus on what you are about to say.

IF POSSIBLE, BE AS SPECIFIC AS YOU CAN: This isn't easy, and it may be better for you to take it in stages. For example, you might *start* with some generalities, like, "Can we talk about what's going on at the moment?" That may make it easier to follow up with, "For the last couple of days, I've really been wondering about...."

In that way, you'll ease your way into important topics, and your listener will be drawn into focusing on what it is you want or need.

CHECK THAT YOUR MESSAGE IS BEING RECEIVED: It's a good idea to break up your own speech with little phrases or queries to check that the other person understands what you're saying: "Do you see what I mean?" or "Does that make sense to you?" or the more universal "Are you with me?"

DO A SHORT RECAP AT THE END: Make sure that what you've said has been heard. If you have asked for some things to be done, for example, it's worth summarizing, "So you'll call your mother about next weekend, and also ask Dorothy to collect the children on Friday."

YOU ARE ALLOWED TO TALK ABOUT OTHER THINGS AS WELL! After you've covered the main topics, don't feel embarrassed to go back to small talk: "Let's talk about some other things now." As someone once remarked, small talk is the mortar of human communication. It's true: the heavy bricks of important issues would soon fall without normal human nattering acting as mortar between them.

HUMOR: As I said above, if humor was useful to you before you were ill, it will be useful to you now. Humor is a coping strategy. It helps the user to draw a frame around something that is threatening and, by laughing at it, to reduce its importance and the size of the threat.

If humor has been part of the way you have coped with threatening crises in the past, it will help you now, and you needn't be afraid of its effects.

If on the other hand you have not used humor as part of your armaments in the past, this may not be a good time to start doing so (despite what Norman Cousins implied in his book *Anatomy of an Illness*).

These guidelines will, I hope, help you keep a conversation relatively comfortable. Now let's discuss how you can bring your own feelings into the conversation.

"How Can I Talk about My Feelings?"

Despite the impression you get from Hollywood movies, most of us are not very good at talking about how we feel. We are not accustomed to it and if we try it, we often feel awkward. Most of the time that doesn't matter. But when something serious happens, such as an illness and particularly a diagnosis of a cancer, most people find that although they want to talk about how they feel, they are not used to it, and they can't. This, by the way, is completely normal!

The Key Is to Acknowledge Every Strong Emotion

Now the first point about expressing feelings is that if you or your listener has strong emotions that are not talked about, you won't be able to talk about any subject easily. An emotion that nobody acknowledges—not mentioning "the elephant in the room"—has a paralyzing effect on all conversation.

So if you are feeling, say, angry or embarrassed or very sad, or if your listener is feeling one of those emotions, then until one of you acknowledges that fact *by mentioning it*, your conversation will feel very sticky. Both of you will be preoccupied and neither of you will be listening.

The moment one of you acknowledges the emotion—"I'm sorry I'm in such a bad mood today, but I've just been told that..."—you will suddenly find communication much easier. Acknowledging, by mentioning, the existence of an emotion partly neutralizes the paralyzing effect that it would otherwise have.

Here's how it's done:

THE SIMPLEST WAY OF ACKNOWLEDGING IS A TECHNIQUE CALLED THE EMPATHIC RESPONSE, and it's actually quite simple. It consists of three straightforward steps:

a. *identify your emotion*—give a name to what you are feeling, for example, anger, sadness, frustration;
b. *identify the cause* of that feeling—bad news that you've just heard, or not being able to go home when you expected; and
c. *acknowledge* the emotion by linking *a* and *b*.

For example, if you are feeling worried because you are waiting for a test result, a good empathic response might be something like, "I'm really worried at the moment because they said I'd have the test result by now and I haven't heard yet."

An empathic response—by acknowledging the feelings that are "in the room"—is always better than trying to ignore your worry, or snapping at the other person because they're late.

The beauty of making an empathic response is that by doing it you are *describing* your feelings rather than simply *displaying* them, *explaining* them rather than simply *exhibiting* them. There's a great deal of difference between saying, "I'm feeling really angry today because..." which starts a conversation, and showing your anger by being curt or rude, which stops conversation.

REMEMBER THAT YOU ARE PERFECTLY ENTITLED TO FEEL ANY WAY YOU LIKE! The way you feel is the way you feel. Emotions are not right or wrong. It is only when you try to cover up any strong feelings that problems really become hard to solve.

DON'T BE AFRAID TO TELL THE OTHER PERSON HOW MUCH SHE OR HE MEANS TO YOU. Again, in our daily lives we don't often do that. But when there is a crisis, it's really worthwhile explaining to the other person how you feel about them.

IF YOU ARE UNCERTAIN ABOUT SOMETHING (ANYTHING!), YOU CAN SAY SO. Don't be afraid to acknowledge uncertainties. If you don't know how you feel, or if you don't know what is going to happen or how you are going to cope, you should say so. More harm is done by pretending that you do know, than is done by confirming that you don't.

THERE ARE MANY OCCASIONS WHEN WORDS AREN'T NEEDED. Holding someone's hand or hugging or simply sitting together in silence can often achieve as much or more than words, once you are both clear about the situation.

EVERYBODY HAS SOME REGRETS IN THEIR LIFE, DESPITE WHAT IT SAYS IN POP SONGS! Don't feel that you are not allowed to express regret. More than any other emotion, regret is reduced when it is shared, and may even prove a durable bond between you and you listener.

NEVER BE AFRAID TO CRY. This is a very important point to remember. Crying is not a sign of weakness, it's a sign of sensitivity and of the emotions you feel. Almost everyone will feel flattered that you feel close enough to them to cry in front of them. So if you do feel like crying, don't think that you have to bottle it all up.

How to Respond to Other People's Reactions

Strangely enough, even though you are the person facing the diagnosis of cancer, you may have more difficulty in dealing with your friend's emotions than with your own. The techniques that I've just described for talking about your own feelings work just as well with the feelings of others.

It's important to be able to deal with emotions, yours or the other person's, because people tend to avoid any emotional situation if they think that somebody can't handle it. In other words, your friend might be tempted to stay away from you rather than face the fact that he or she has strong emotions but doesn't know how to deal with them. It shouldn't be like that, but it often is.

So here's how to use the same techniques to respond to your friend's emotions:

USE THE EMPATHIC RESPONSE: Follow the same three steps to try to acknowledge your friend's feelings. If you are a good guesser, then the ideal is to identify your friend's emotion and what caused it. This can be as simple as, "You look as if you're feeling really uneasy when I talk about the cancer," or "I guess coming here makes you very upset."

YOU CAN USE THE EMPATHIC RESPONSE WITH ANY EMOTION IN THE ROOM: Don't be afraid to acknowledge how you feel at the same time: "This is making both of us feel awful," or "I know you're worried about what's going to happen next and so am I." The more you are each aware of both your own feelings and each other's, the better the dialogue will be.

IF YOU GET INTO SOME FORM OF CONFLICT (and that happens quite often) see Hints for Resolving Conflict on page 189.

How to Tell Other People What's Going On

Many people find it awkward and embarrassing to break the news that there is something medically wrong with them. They all tend to shy away from it. They probably haven't had any practice in doing it and feel that they don't know where to begin.

If the other person is your spouse or partner or a close friend, then it is usually possible to have her or him present when your doctor talks to you. That way, you both hear the same thing. If it happens that your friend cannot be present, then you may find the following guidelines useful is telling her or him the news.

TRY TO GET THE PHYSICAL SETTING RIGHT. That means make sure that the television is turned off, for example, and that you can each look at the other person's face easily.

IT'S ALWAYS WORTH INTRODUCING THE SUBJECT, rather than starting off baldly. Something like, "I think it would be best if I tell you what's going on. Is that OK?"

IF YOU THINK YOUR FRIEND KNOWS SOME OF WHAT HAS BEEN HAPPENING, then it can be quite useful to ask about that, so you don't go over ground that has already been covered. "You probably know some of this already, so why don't you tell me what you make of the situation so far, then I'll take it from there."

IT OFTEN HELPS TO START WITH A PRELIMINARY STATEMENT, a warning shot. For example, if the situation is serious, you can actually say "Well, it sounds as if it might be serious." If the situation is worrying but sounds as if it will be all right in the long term, then say just that.

GIVE THE INFORMATION IN SMALL CHUNKS, a few sentences at a time, and check to make sure—"Do you see what I mean?"—your friend understands what you're saying before you continue.

THERE WILL OFTEN BE SILENCES. Don't be put off by them. You or your friend may well find that just holding hands or sitting together in the same room says more than any words. If you find that a silence makes you feel uncomfortable, the easiest way to break it is with a simple question, "What are you thinking about?"

WHEN YOU TELL SOMEONE CLOSE TO YOU THAT SOMETHING SERIOUS IS WRONG WITH YOU, YOUR FRIEND MAY FEEL SAD AND DEPRESSED, in sympathy with your situation. As a result, you may feel that you ought to put a positive and upbeat spin on the explanation in order to relieve your friend's feelings. If the facts of your situation support a positive spin, then do it. But if there is a great deal of uncertainty or worry about the future, you shouldn't feel that you need to disguise that in order not to hurt anyone's feelings. In other words, try to stay as close to the real situation as you can. It may be painful for your friend at this particular moment, but if you paint a rosy picture that then doesn't materialize, your friend will be much more disappointed (and perhaps more hurt) later on.

You'll find that these principles will make what is always a difficult conversation a bit less awkward. As we've already said, it's not really fair that you should have to do so much, particularly at a time when your own needs are so great. But it often happens like that, and in this way your friend will be much better equipped to give you support in the future.

Talking with Children

Talking with children about your illness, or about their illness if they happen to be the patient, is extremely difficult. We think of childhood as a time of innocence and freedom from pain or guilt. We all hope that unpleasant or painful facts will never intrude into the lives of children until they are older and have adequate coping skills. Unfortunately, serious illness does not respect age. Often, patients do need to tell their children what is happening. Telling a child is often the most awkward and painful part of the illness, but the following guidelines may help you somewhat:

PITCH THE INFORMATION AT THE LEVEL OF THE CHILD'S UNDERSTANDING, NOT THE CHILD'S AGE. Children differ enormously in what they can understand and what they can't. Some five-year-olds can understand concepts that escape other children of ten. So check as you go along to see what the child understands, and tailor what you say to that.

BE PREPARED TO REPEAT THE INFORMATION. Children usually ask for important information to be repeated, perhaps several times. If the subject is painful to you, then you may be tempted to stop the conversation. "I've answered that three times already. That's enough now!" But when children ask for repetition, it's not because they are stupid or malicious, they simply need to check that you really meant what you said. So try to be more patient than usual and go over the ground again, being consistent with what you said last time.

BE AWARE OF WHAT IS KNOWN AS MAGICAL THINKING. Children almost always feel very guilty when things go wrong around them, and often feel that in some undefined way they are to blame for the situation. This is called *magical thinking*: "If I'd cleaned up my room when Mommy told me to, she wouldn't be ill now." So it's really worth making sure that children understand that the situation is not their fault. It's often worth building that into an overall statement such as, "This is just one of those bad things that happen occasionally and it's nobody's fault. It's not my fault, it's not the doctor's fault and it's certainly not your fault. It's just a piece of really bad luck."

ASK YOURSELF IF YOU WOULD LIKE SOME HELP. Very often, having a health-care professional present can be very helpful. I have conducted many interviews like this, and it is helpful because the child can often focus any anger or resentment on the professional, instead of on the parent. The professional becomes a sort of lightning conductor, and that may reduce the burden on you. Also there may be questions which are difficult technically to answer. The professional can help you there too.

So it is worth asking your healthcare team if there is a doctor or a nurse or a therapist or social worker or anyone else who might help.

Explaining difficult or threatening facts to a child is always painful. These guidelines may help a bit, but don't hesitate to ask for whatever other help is available to you.

Hints for Resolving Conflict

When the diagnosis is cancer, the emotional atmosphere is fraught, and conflict is common. It may be conflict with your friends or family or, more likely, with some member of your healthcare team.

Many patients find themselves getting particularly and almost uncontrollably cross or angry with friends or the healthcare team. Some of this feeling is generated by the basic human reaction of blaming the messenger for the message. When somebody tells you that you have a cancer, you find it difficult to focus your anger on the cancer itself so you focus it on the person who told you.

This reaction is often heightened by the feeling that you have the misfortune to have a disease and the other person seems to be getting away scot-free.

In all events, it is quite possible that there will be conflict at some stage between you and somebody else, and here are some guidelines that will help you to resolve some of the areas of conflict, insofar as they are resolvable.

WHENEVER POSSIBLE, try to *describe* your feelings rather than *display* them. As emotions rise, try to acknowledge those emotions—whether they are yours or the other person's.

TRY TO DISINVEST IN THE OUTCOME OF THE ARGUMENT. In other words try—and it's not easy—not to feel that your worth as a human being is tied to the outcome of the dispute. It's easy to imagine that if you win, you are a wonderful person, and if you lose you are not. But that is not true, as almost every conflict known to humankind has shown. So tell yourself that you are still a perfectly wonderful person, even if you lose this argument.

IF THERE IS AN ISSUE OR AN AREA OVER WHICH YOU CANNOT AGREE, try to define that area even though you can't resolve it. In other words, "agree to disagree" on that particular issue.

TALK THE DISPUTE OVER WITH SOMEONE ELSE. And as you describe it, try not to turn the other party in the dispute into a monster. Go even farther: try to "de-monstrify" the other person as you describe the dispute. That way, you may see a way out of the argument simply by describing it from one step back.

Talking with the Person with a Cancer Diagnosis (Tips for Friends and Family)

This section of Part Four is intended specifically for the friend or family member, and in it I set out a few basic guidelines of how to listen, and a systematic strategy for listening and talking. (Note that some issues and topics in this section repeat what was said in the previous section. I am assuming that most readers will read one or the other, but if you happen to read both, there will be some repetition. I apologize in advance.)

Not Knowing What to Say

We all feel awkward when a friend receives some bad news, even if things later work out much better than we at first feared. Usually, and especially if the bad news is a cancer diagnosis, *we don't know what to say*.

To make things worse we often think there are things we *should* be saying or doing that would automatically make things easier for the person with a cancer, if only we knew what they were.

In fact, that's not true.

There is no best thing or correct thing that you should be saying: what matters most is not what you say, but how you listen.

So let's start with the assumption that your friend has had a diagnosis of cancer and that you want to be of help and support, but you don't know how. (All of the following hints and guidelines are summarized in a handy *aide-mémoire*—the s.c.a.n.s strategy—at the end of this section on page 196.)

How to Be a Good Listener

Basically, good listening can be divided into two parts—physical and mental. A lot of the most awkward communication gaps are caused by not knowing a few simple rules which encourage free conversation.

GET THE SETTING RIGHT. The *physical context* is important, and it's a good idea to get the details correct at the start. Get comfortable, sit down, try to look relaxed (even if you don't feel it), try to signal the fact that you are there to spend some time (for instance, take your coat off).

Keep your *eyes on the same level* as the person you're talking to, which almost always means sitting down. As a general rule, if your friend is in hospital and chairs are unavailable or too low, sitting on the bed is preferable to standing—as long as you have the patient's permission first. (For the hospital patient, the bed is the entire extent of home territory—nobody should invade it by sitting down without asking permission first.)

In other circumstances, you should try to keep the atmosphere as private as possible. Don't try to talk in a corridor, for example, or on a staircase. That seems obvious, but actual conversations often go wrong because of these simple things. So, try to create the right space, although however hard you try, there will always be interruptions—phones ringing, doorbells sounding, children coming in, and so on. You can only do your best.

Keep within a comfortable distance of the patient. Generally there should be one to two feet of space between you. A longer distance makes dialogue feel awkward and formal, and a shorter distance can make your friend feel hemmed in, particularly if he or she is in bed and unable to back away. Make sure there are no physical obstacles (desks, bedside tables, and so on) between you. Again, that may not be easy, but if you say something like, "It's not very easy to talk across this table, can I move it aside for a moment?" it helps both of you.

Keep looking at your friend, no matter which one of you is talking. Eye contact is what tells the other person that a conversation is solely between the two of you. If, during a painful moment, you can't look directly at each other, at least stay close and hold the person's hand or touch them if you can.

FIND OUT WHETHER YOUR FRIEND WANTS TO TALK. The other person may simply not be in the mood to talk, or may not want to talk to you that day. Try not to be offended if that's the case. If you're not sure, you can always ask, "Do you feel like talking?" This is always better than launching into a deep conversation, "Tell me about your feelings," when a patient is tired or has just been talking to someone else.

SHOW THAT YOU'RE LISTENING WHILE YOU LISTEN. When your friend is talking, you should try to do two things: listen to what's being said instead of thinking of what you're going to say next, and *show* that you're listening.

To listen properly, you must be thinking about what your friend is saying. You should not be rehearsing your reply. Doing that would mean that you're anticipating what you think is *about* to be said, and not listening to what they *is* being said. And try not to interrupt. While she is talking, don't talk yourself, but wait for her to stop speaking before you start. If she interrupts you while you're saying something with a "but..." or an "I thought..." or something similar, you should stop and let her speak.

ENCOURAGE THE OTHER PERSON TO TALK. Good listening isn't just sitting there like a running tape recorder. You can actually help the patient talk about what's on his mind by *encouraging* him. Simple things work very well. Try nodding, or saying affirmative things like "Yes" or "I see" or "Tell me more." Those all sound simple, but at times of maximum stress it's the simple things you need to help you along.

You can also show that you're hearing, and listening, by *repeating* one or two words from the patient's last sentence. This really does help him to feel that his words are being understood. When medical students are shown this technique, they invariably report that using it at home with their friends and family members always moves the conversation along and makes the listener suddenly appear more interested and involved.

You can also *reflect* back to the talker what you've heard—partly to check that you've got it right, and partly to show that you're listening and trying to understand. You can say things like, "So you mean that..." or "If I've got that straight, you feel..." or even "I hear you," although that last one might sound a bit self-conscious if it isn't your usual style.

DON'T FORGET SILENCE AND NONVERBAL COMMUNICATION. If someone stops talking, it usually means that she or he is thinking about something painful or sensitive. Wait with your friend for a moment. Hold his hand or rest your hand on her arm, if you feel like it. Then ask what he or she was thinking about. Don't rush it, although silences at emotional moments do seem to last for years.

During a silence, sometimes you may think, "I have no idea what to say." On occasion, this may be because there isn't anything *to* say. If that's the case, don't be afraid to say nothing and just stay close. At times like that, a touch or an arm around the patient's shoulder can be of greater value than anything you say.

Sometimes, nonverbal communication tells you much more about the other person than you might have expected

DON'T BE AFRAID TO DESCRIBE YOUR OWN FEELINGS. You are allowed to say things like, "I find this difficult to talk about." or "I'm not very good at talking about…" or even "I don't know what to say." Medical students are often taught this when they learn communication skills. As one of them reported back to me, "I tried what you told me, telling the patient that I found it awkward, and it *really worked*." That student was pleasantly surprised. You will be too.

CLARIFY. Make sure you haven't misunderstood.

If you are sure you understand what your friend means, you can say so. Responses such as "You sound very low," or "That must have made you very angry," are replies that tell her that you've picked up the emotions she has been talking about or showing. But if you're not sure what the patient means, then ask, "What did that feel like?" or "What do you think of it?" or "How do you feel now?" Misunderstandings can arise if you make assumptions and are wrong.

It's certainly advantageous when you instinctively pick up what a friend is feeling, but if you don't happen to do that, don't hesitate to ask. Something like, "Help me understand what you mean a bit more," is useful.

DON'T CHANGE THE SUBJECT. If your friend wants to talk about how rotten he feels, let him do exactly that. It may be difficult for you to hear some of the things he is saying, but if you can manage it, then stay with him while he talks. If you find it too uncomfortable and think you can't handle the conversation at that moment, then you should say so, and offer to discuss it again later. You can even say very simple and obvious things like, "This is making me feel very uncomfortable at the moment. Can we come back to it later?" Don't simply change the subject without acknowledging the fact that your friend has raised it.

DON'T OFFER ADVICE PREMATURELY. Ideally, no one should give advice to anyone else unless it's asked for. However, this isn't an ideal world and quite often we find ourselves doing just that. Try not to give advice early in the conversation, because it stops dialogue. If you're bursting to give advice it's often easier to use phrases like, "Have you thought about trying…" or "A friend of mine once tried…" Those are both less bald than "If I were you I'd…" which makes the patient think, or even say, "But you're not me." And that really is a conversation stopper.

RESPOND TO HUMOR. Many people can't imagine there could be anything to laugh about if you are facing a serious illness or threat to health. However, as I've pointed out before, humor actually serves an important function in coping with major threats and fears.

Humor allows us to *ventilate*, to get rid of intense feelings, and to get things into perspective. Humor is one of the ways human beings deal with things that seem impossible. The most common subjects of jokes include mothers-in-law, fear of flying, hospitals and doctors, and sex. None of those subjects is intrinsically funny. An argument with a mother-in-law can be very distressing for everyone concerned, but arguing with your mother-in-law has been an easy laugh for the stand-up comedian for decades, because we all laugh most easily at the things we cope with least easily.

We laugh at things to get them into perspective, to reduce them in size and threat. And if your friend uses humor as part of a coping strategy, then don't hesitate to respond to it. It will help him or her to cope and reinforce the bond between the two if you.

And, finally, here is the summary that I promised.

The S.C.A.N.S Mnemonic: An Aide-Mémoire for Effective Listening

Setting. Get the setting right. Sit down, eyes on same level as other person, and look as "at ease" as you can.

Communication Skills. Don't talk over the other person. Keep quiet while the other person talks. Use simple techniques such as nodding, smiling, and using one word from their last sentence in your first sentence (which demonstrates that you were listening).

Acknowledgment. Always acknowledge the existence of the other person's emotion(s) if it's intense; for example, "It must be very frustrating having to wait for the results."

Negotiating. Clarify what it is that the other person wants—practical, informational, or emotional. Then clarify what it is that you can do and are good at. Then do the things on your list that seem to fit the other person's list.

Summary. Always end a discussion by summarizing the main two or three points that you've been talking about together. Ask if there are other important issues. End with a clear "contract," which can be as simple as, "I'll see you on Friday," or "I'll phone you next week."

"How Can I Help?"–A Checklist for Friends

The real problem is knowing what to do first.

Here is a very handy checklist to guide you in the practical details of helping a friend:

1. MAKE YOUR OFFER. You must first find out whether or not your help is *wanted*. If there are other people involved in support, you should find out whether your help is *needed*, and if it is, make your offer. Your initial offer should be specific. Don't say, "Let me know if there's anything I can do." Say clearly that you'll check back to see if there are things you can help with. Obviously if you are the parent or the spouse, you don't need to ask. But in most other circumstances it is important to know whether you are in the right position to help. Sometimes a distant acquaintance or colleague is more welcome than a close relative, so don't prejudge your usefulness. Do not be upset if the patient does not seem to want your support. Don't take it personally. If you are still keen to help, see if there are other family members who need assistance. After you have made your initial offer, do not wait to be called, but check back with a few preliminary suggestions, such as "Do you want me to mow the grass?" or "Can I pick up some groceries for you?"

2. BECOME INFORMED, BUT NOT A WORLD EXPERT. If you are to be useful to your friend, you will need some information about the medical situation, but only enough to make sensible plans. You do not need to, and *should not*, become a world expert on the subject. Many helpers are drawn to acquire more and more details which are not necessarily relevant to their particular friend's situation. Sometimes their motive is curiosity, sometimes it is a desire to be in control.

3. ASSESS THE NEEDS. This means assessing the needs of both the patient and the rest of the family. Naturally, any assessment is going to be full of uncertainties because the future is often unpredictable, but you should think about the patient's needs. These will vary with how disabling the disease is at any one time (if it is disabling at all, of course). If the patient is seriously inconvenienced then here are some of the questions you might ask yourself: Who is going to look after him during the

day? Can she get from bed to toilet by herself? Can he prepare his own meals? Does she need medications that she cannot take herself?

And of the other family members, ask yourself: Are there children that need to be taken to and from school? Is the spouse medically fit or are there things the spouse needs too? Is the home suitable for the patient's medical condition, or are there things that need to be done there? Any list will be long and almost certainly incomplete, but it is a start. Check your list by going through a day in the life of your friend and thinking what will be needed at each stage.

4. DECIDE WHAT YOU CAN DO AND WANT TO DO. What are you good at? Can you cook for the patient? (For instance, delivering precooked frozen meals is always welcome.) Can you prepare meals for other family members? Are you handy around the house? Could you put up handrails or wheelchair ramps if required? Could you house-sit, so that the spouse can visit the patient? Could you take the kids to the zoo for the day to give the couple some time together?

If you aren't good at any of these things, would you be prepared to pay for, say, a cleaner for a half-day a week to help out? Could you locate relevant booklets for the patient? Can you find videos that the patient likes? Does the patient need the furniture rearranged? (For instance, your friend may need to sleep on the ground floor because she cannot manage stairs.) Perhaps you could arrange some colorful bouquets of flowers in the house on the day your friend gets out of hospital?

5. START WITH SMALL PRACTICAL THINGS. Look at the list of the things you can do and are prepared to do, and start by offering a few of them. Don't offer all of them at once. This will overwhelm the patient. Pick some small items that are practical that the patient might not be able to do easily. Making a small "contract" and fulfilling it is far better than aiming too high and failing.

It may require a little creative thought and maybe some inside knowledge. For instance, one of my patients used to get his hair cut every week. It wasn't a big thing, but it was part of his regular routine. When he was in hospital, his friend arranged for the hospital barber to call weekly. That was a nice and thoughtful touch, and there are lots of things like that. Another patient was a schoolteacher. Her teaching colleagues got the children to draw cards for her. Again, a small thing, but thoughtful and highly valued by the patient.

6. AVOID EXCESSES. Don't give huge gifts that overwhelm and embarrass. Don't, for instance, buy the patient a new car unless you know specifically that this is wanted and it will not cause embarrassment. Most large gifts spring from a sense of guilt on the part of the donor, and create guilt in the recipient. Similarly, your offers of help should be modest and suited to the patient and family. Be sensitive.

7. LISTEN. Time is a present you can always give. If you haven't already done so, have a look at the guidelines above on sensitive listening, and try to spend regular time with your friend. Don't spend two hours once a month, unless you cannot do any more, of course. It's better to spend ten or fifteen minutes once a day or every couple of days if you can. Be reliable: visit your friend when you say you will. As the saying goes, "half of being there for someone is simply being there."

8. INVOLVE OTHER PEOPLE. Be fair to yourself and recognize your own limitations. Every helper and supporter wants to do his or her best, and you may be very tempted to undertake heroic tasks, out of a sense of anger or rage against your friend's situation and the injustice of it. But if you make heroic gestures and then fail, you will become part of the problem instead of part of the solution. You owe it to yourself and to your friend to undertake reasonable tasks so that you succeed. This

means you should always be realistic about what you can do, and get other people to help with what you can't.

Going through this list in your mind is valuable because it offers a genuinely practical approach to something that is probably unfamiliar to you, and because it quells your own sense of panic and not knowing where to start. I've summarized it in the checklist below. Whatever plans you make will certainly change with time, as conditions change. Be prepared to be flexible and learn on the job.

CHECKLIST FOR FRIENDS

I. MAKE YOUR OFFER

Be specific. Do not just say, "Call me if you need anything."

2. BECOME INFORMED ABOUT YOUR FRIEND'S MEDICAL SITUATION

But don't try to become a world expert on it.

3. ASSESS THE NEEDS

A good way is to go mentally through a typical day that you friend is likely to experience.

4. DECIDE WHAT YOU CAN DO AND WHAT YOU WANT TO DO

5. START WITH SMALL PRACTICAL THINGS

You can always cook some frozen meals, or take the children out for an afternoon, etc.

6. AVOID EXCESSES

Inappropriately generous or excessive gifts or gestures are almost worse than doing nothing.

7. YOU CAN ALWAYS SIT AND LISTEN

8. ACCEPT THAT YOU HAVE LIMITATIONS—SO TRY TO INVOLVE OTHER PEOPLE

Why You Matter to Your Friend

Of course the whole situation is scary—for you as well as for your friend. In fact, the only people who aren't frightened may be those who have no imagination at all! But by listening to what your friend is most concerned about and by helping her or him to obtain the right information and understand it, you can be a vital part of the support system. And that is one of the most important things that one human being can do for another.

Spirituality, Religion, and Faith: Benefits and Occasional Problems

Spirituality is a difficult and sometimes touchy subject.

Spirituality is not the same as religion—a great number of people regard themselves as spiritual, but do not think of themselves as religious. Spirituality can be very important in times of crisis, and particularly important in helping you to cope with a threat that may be perceived (whether it is true or not) as life-threatening.

In this section, I'm going to discuss a few of the topics in spirituality that are most commonly raised and discussed: how you can identify and explore the spiritual aspects of your own personality; how to initiate conversations about spiritual aspects, and with whom; what techniques may help you; and how to deal with the rare instances of "bad religiosity," when religious advisors might actually add to your problems rather than helping you solve them.

"What Is Spirituality and How Do I Know How Important It Is to Me?"

We use the words *spiritual* and *spirituality* frequently and easily. When we think about what they describe, however, it's actually quite difficult to put it into words. Although it might seem somewhat out of place in a medical book, I'm going to summarize some of the current thinking about spirituality, and some of the practical issues.

When most people use the word *spirituality* they are usually talking about a state of mind that is different from the ordinary, everyday state of mind in which we function and operate most of the time. They usually have in mind a state in which the person is deeply tranquil and calm, and thinking about or feeling the deeper and more fundamental issues of existence. As one church minister put it, "Spirituality is more about the meaning of a person's existence than about the fact that the price of gas has gone up by three cents a liter." I thought that was a very useful—and practical—handle on a rather amorphous and indefinable subject.

Spirituality refers to those moments in which we are able mentally to step outside of the smaller day-to-day worries and concerns, or even little victories and triumphs, and get in touch with a more central part of our thinking and feeling—a deliberate and gentle plunge into the deeper and unaccustomed waters of ourselves.

Transcendence: The Essence of Spiritual Experience

Another word for this, and it is a word that appears more and more frequently in theological writings these days, is *transcendence*. The word implies a crossing of the daily boundaries, limits, and horizons of our thinking and feeling—an activity that involves going beyond, transcending, the usual concerns of daily living.

The process of achieving a state of spiritual transcendence is not directly related to religious observances. Many people certainly find it easier to get into a more spiritual mode of thinking and feeling when they are in a church or synagogue or temple (or any other place of worship), often when they are surrounded by other people doing the same thing and saying the same words (during a religious service for example). But many other people do not. In fact, some people find themselves noticeably distracted by the other people and all the wide variety of social signals ("What's she wearing?" and "Why didn't he smile at me?")

Where you go to enter into a state or transcendence, or how you do it, is not of major importance. What really matters is that, when you do get into a transcendent state, it brings you a recognizable relief from day-to-day stress and provides you with an oasis of calm.

Transcendence implies coping better. It is not the same as gritting your teeth, or grinning and bearing it. It is more a matter of rolling with the punches. And that is something you can do much more effectively when you tap into your own spiritual resources.

"Whom Should I Talk To?"

The key to getting support from the spiritual elements of your own personality is achieving transcendence. That means achieving a state in which the day-to-day stresses of your cancer and its treatment cause you less discomfort and pain. And that depends more on the type of discussions you have, than it does on the doctrinal and formal aspects of a religion or sect.

In other words, if you know someone—a priest, rabbi, imam, chaplain, chaplaincy student, or counselor, for example—with whom you feel comfortable in discussing spiritual matters and with whom you feel relaxed and closer to a state of transcendence, then my advice is: go for it. Ask them to sit down and discuss the questions that are bothering you.

If you find that you get that sense of comfort from being in a church or temple, and that you like the sense of community that you get there, but you are in hospital at the moment, tell the chaplain. If there is a chapel in the hospital (and nowadays there is quite likely to be a multi-faith place of worship) plan a visit if you are able.

In my opinion, a really good person to talk to is even better than a really good religion.

"What Should I Do?"

The answer to the question, "What should I do?" is simple: do whatever works to get you into a calmer and more tranquil state. If you gain strength and calm from saying prayers, listening to sacred music, or reading religious texts, do it. If you are able to practice meditation, do that. (If you want to learn how to meditate, there are dozens of books that will teach you quite quickly.)

Whatever works to get you into that private and refreshing and renewing space, do it.

Bad Religiosity

I have one caution however: very occasionally you may come across religious people who pursue their own particular doctrine with an uncaring, heartless, and even punitive zeal and energy. I once encountered a priest of a strange fundamentalist sect who told a patient that her sufferings were God's way of preparing her for the much worse sufferings that she was going to experience in Hell!

Incidents like this are extremely rare these days, but they happen occasionally. There are a few people who take advantage of a patient's vulnerability and threatened health to gain doctrinal or sectarian converts. I think this is totally unscrupulous, and very far from the ideal and principle of every religion in the world.

So if you find that your spiritual advisor is actually increasing your anxiety and your sense of psychological and spiritual discomfort, then discontinue those discussions and find someone else to talk to.

"Does Intercessionary Prayer Change the Course of a Disease?"

Finally, I want to deal with an issue that has been prominent for many years, and on which research has recently provided a definitive answer. The question is whether or not having people pray for you can actually make your medical condition better.

When any member of a community is ill, it is very common for the local priest or religious leader to ask members of the congregation to remember that person in their prayers and thoughts. This, I believe, is a good and supportive action, and when people are told that the congregation is doing that, it often gives them a feeling of being supported and being in touch with their community, even if they're physically absent (in hospital, for example).

Recently, however, the idea developed that there was a scientific basis to this activity and that intercessionary prayer (prayer to God, or gods, by other people) could actually change the course of a disease. What started that particular ball rolling was a paper by a Dr. William Byrd whose data suggested that people who were prayed for after a heart attack (without being informed of it themselves) spent less time in hospital than people who were not prayed for, although they did not live longer or suffer fewer consequences of the heart attack.

The controversy over this was immense. It seemed theologically unsound that a god would allow prayed-for heart attack patients to go home from hospital earlier, but still to suffer the same number of heart-rhythm disturbances, and second heart attacks, and actually not to live longer than unprayed-for patients.

The discussions were intense and prolonged, and eventually a study was set up to test this hypothesis. The results, published in the *Lancet* in 2005, showed no such effect on the process of recovery from a heart attack. Being the subject of "passive prayer" does *not* mysteriously affect the course of heart disease. And conversely anyone who happens *not* to be prayed for is not missing out.

Sex and Sexuality: Problems and Strategies

Sex is a subject that is discussed only rarely during clinic or office visits. Lack of time, embarrassment, and social taboos make it difficult for us to talk easily and honestly about sex.

In this section, I offer a few hints and guidelines that may make this awkward topic a little less difficult to talk about.

Sex as Antidote

The sexual urge is a powerful one for the majority of people. In fact, it is one of the few urges powerful enough to be an antidote to pain and misery, at least some of the time. For patients, sex may sometimes be the only readily accessible means of escape, albeit temporary, from the world of worry and misery that seems to enclose them. Furthermore, sex is not only a means of escape, it is also a route to human contact and intimacy. Because it is a normal activity, it may also be an important way to help the patient feel like a normal human being.

The Many Sources of Difficulty

For most couples, sexuality is a fairly fragile thing that even in the daily run of life can be upset by a wide range of things, including arguments, stress, and worry. Even in times of perfect health, then, the multiple sources of stress and conflict can make things really difficult. But the situation is almost always a lot worse in the face of any long-term illness or threat of illness.

Above and beyond the everyday stresses and strains, a serious illness can, and almost always does, affect your sex life badly.

PSYCHOLOGICAL FACTORS: Even if both partners are feeling completely well physically, the many anxieties triggered by the cancer diagnosis itself—and all the worries that come with it: about the future, about coping, about work, about treatment, about the children, about finances, and so on—can put you off your game.

PHYSICAL FACTORS: In addition to the psychological stresses, there may be physical problems as well. General physical symptoms such as pain or nausea can affect both the libido (the desire to initiate sex) or the performance or both. Headache (from any cause) is often made worse when the intracranial pressure rises during sex.

As well as the general problems, and depending on the site of a cancer and the type of treatment, there may also be specific physical problems which affect sexual activity directly. For example, after surgery or radiotherapy to the pelvis, there may be pain on penetration (the medical term is *dyspareunia*), soreness, and difficulties with lubrication. Erectile dysfunction is common after prostate surgery or radiotherapy as well. Urinary catheters or conditions affecting the back or hips, a stoma, and hair loss after chemotherapy can have a similar effect. Any of these may impede or prevent a couple from having sex when they wish.

PERCEIVED ATTRACTIVENESS: Furthermore there are often secondary psychological problems associated with the changes in appearance following surgery.

Many operations produce some change in appearance, but mastectomy and colostomies are common examples, and both may make the patient feel unattractive to the partner, and ashamed. Often this causes the partner to feel uncertain about how to reassure the patient, even when—as is often the case—the partner's physical attraction to the patient is not actually diminished.

The Taboos

For most of us, for a lot of the time, sexuality is much more than a physical issue.

For many people, sex is an extremely important component of their relationships but is a subject that is rarely talked about openly and candidly. And for most of the time, this does not matter. But when a serious illness affects one partner, then it does matter.

In fact, specialists in this subject have found that sexual problems are almost universal among cancer patients who were sexually active at the time of diagnosis. Most of us in the healthcare professions did not realize how common these problems were because we didn't ask!

Stress is often a culprit. Obviously the diagnosis of cancer in one partner is going to affect the relationship in a major way. It may be the biggest strain ever put upon the relationship up to that point. There is the fear of the disease, the fear of the treatment, the uncertainty about the future, and many other important factors. Just like any major stress, such as unemployment or bereavement, these may seriously and adversely affect sexual libido, in either the patient or the partner or both. Further, depression very commonly decreases sexual libido. In fact, loss of interest in sex is one of the hallmarks and diagnostic features of depression.

Specific Interpersonal Problems

In addition to the physical problems and to general stress, there are many other factors. In any relationship, one or more of these factors may turn out to be significant:

SOCIAL AND STATUS CHANGES. Chronic illness of any sort—particularly if the future is somewhat uncertain—may result in the patient being put on disability insurance, for example. If the patient was formerly the breadwinner of the family, then this change may have marked psychological fallout, and may cause considerable tension between the partners.

OTHER INTERPERSONAL ISSUES. If, between the two partners, there are other issues that may have been only partly resolved and may have lain dormant before the illness, these issues may now surface and create tension. The attitude of either partner to illness itself, to the possibility of dying, to religious factors, to ways of dealing with physical symptoms within the relationship are examples of the types of issues that may surface. Also, the partner might fear hurting the patient during sex, or even fear catching the cancer.

There are, therefore, a range of factors that may affect sex within the relationship and may stop most sexual activity altogether. This requires attention, so that it does not undermine most of the other aspects of the relationship.

Getting Sex Started Again

Starting sex again is never easy.

Quite often you feel awkward, embarrassed, and unfamiliar in the new circumstances. And these feelings may be heightened by the memories of what your sex life used to be like, and (sometimes) by the feeling that somehow you ought to be able to recreate your previous sex life immediately.

If this is what the patient wants—and it may be or may not be—then it is very important that you both try to discuss it. If you do not, the patient will feel rejected and isolated. As one of my patients put it, "For a time I was a sexual pariah."

You may find that the following guidelines provide a practical approach to getting sex started again.

YOU MUST TALK ABOUT IT. In my experience, somebody facing an illness such as a cancer usually wants intimacy and human contact even more than sexual gratification itself. So if one of you cannot actually manage to join in sex, then do not make up an excuse. Making up a spurious excuse will simply add an air of dishonesty to an already tense situation. You should be prepared to talk about it, and to listen. If you feel tender toward the other person and want to be intimate but cannot show those feelings sexually, then it is really important and helpful to say so. Very often, that expression of tenderness and concern will help in itself.

MAKE PLANS. Making and discussing plans about sex is something that most of us do not normally do: most of the time we don't have to. When there is an illness, however, you may have to do that, however awkward and embarrassing it is at first. You should try to be quite specific about what you can do and are prepared to do. Often a cuddle or a hug will achieve a great deal and, if you have discussed it in advance, will not cause feelings of distrust or guilt if things go no further at that time.

One of the most common problems is what to do if the patient is in hospital. A decade ago, most hospital authorities had a pretty clear idea about what couples were supposed to do about intimacy in a hospital: nothing. Nowadays, most hospitals will allow a couple some privacy, so do not be afraid to ask.

Other problems that you can sort out include where you both should sleep. If the patient has physical symptoms that cause disturbance in sleep, then it may be easier for you to sleep in separate beds for part of the night. Again, if you talk about this you will find that it need not lead to feelings of rejection or guilt.

TAKE ONE STEP AT A TIME. Particularly if you had a healthy sex life before the illness, you might think that you ought to be able to get right back to a normal sex life. Usually that will not happen, and if you are expecting it you might feel discouraged. Do not be afraid to take it slowly. Start with simple cuddles or hugs, increasing gradually to a greater range of sexual activities. Also be aware that physical problems might make it important for you to change the positions of sexual intercourse. This also requires discussion, planning, and a gradual approach.

GET HELP IF YOU NEED IT. You may find that you cannot make progress in addressing sexual problems. If that happens, do not be afraid to ask for help. There are sexual counselors available, and a small amount of counseling and help can make a huge difference.

Sex is one of the most important components in many relationships. When it goes wrong, it needs a lot of discussion and dialogue to start the process of restoring it. The secret is to talk about it (and not, as it were, to turn your back on the problem), to accept that progress may be slow and intermittent, and not to be afraid of getting professional help if you need it.

Hope: How to Have It and How to Handle It

"You must never take away hope." It's a time-honored saying. Everyone has heard it, and most people believe it. The real challenge, however, is how to maintain hope while still making realistic plans in case things don't go well.

Nothing I say in this section will diminish the importance of hope, in everyone's daily life, whether they are ill or not. But we do need to look in greater detail at what hope is and how it functions for everyone, every day.

In that way we will be able to see how hope can often help us to deal with threatening situations, but also how it can sometimes be counter-productive and may interfere with the making of practical plans.

"What Is Hope Anyway?"

Hope is not a monolith: it is not a single indivisible entity or thing. Hope is the expectation of a positive outcome when that outcome is not yet known.

In other words, hope is a feeling that we experience, when we are in a developing situation with an unknown outcome, that it will all work out well. Hope is therefore an emotion, associated with the expectation of a positive, beneficial conclusion. Hope is the feeling we get in anticipation of a happy ending.

In itself, hope can be an enormous help to us. Hope can give us motivation, energy, and strength to face up to and deal with difficult circumstances. But it can also disable our abilities to make practical "what if" plans, to prepare a Plan B in case things do not work out well.

This ambiguity of hope—potentially both helpful and unhelpful—was brilliantly illustrated by the Cornell physician Eric Cassell, author of *The Meaning of Suffering* and many other works on the philosophy of medicine. In a lecture entitled "Hope as an Enemy," Dr. Cassell used the analogy of running to catch a plane to focus on the potential dangers of relying on hope, alone and exclusively, instead of making backup plans as well. (This version is paraphrased from the original.)

Imagine that I'm running down the concourse of an airport to catch the nine o'clock flight to Toronto, and it's already five minutes past nine and I'm still two minutes away from the gate.

Am I crazy to be running? And to be hoping that I'll make the flight? Well, of course not.

It can happen that there's a delay, and boarding starts late, so that even if you're a few minutes late arriving at the gate you just might be okay (as actually happened this morning). Also, I'm not crazy because as I'm running, I know that in my pocket I've got a timetable of all the other flights that leave for Toronto, including one at ten o'clock. Furthermore, I've got the kind of ticket that can be changed easily.

But what if I'm running down the concourse already late for the nine o'clock flight, and I've got a nonrefundable ticket that can't be changed at all, and I have no idea of how I will get to Toronto if I miss the nine o'clock flight?

And what if the time now is not five past nine, but half-past eleven? Or nine o'clock on the following day? What then?

If that's the situation, am I crazy to be running?

Cassell's point is that the act of running—the embodiment of hoping—is not crazy *in itself*. It is an important human activity and also, depending on the circumstances, the object of the hope may happen. However, it *is* counterproductive, and may actually make your situation worse, if hope is the *only* thing you do. If you fail to make plans as well.

Another friend of mine, an accountant, had his own analogy.

If you ask people how they are planning to pay their income tax this year and they say, "Oh, I've paid most of it by installments during the year and I've set aside a bit for April," you know that they are looking after themselves well. But if they say, "Income tax? Well, I bought a lottery ticket and I'm certain that I'm going to win before April," then you really do worry about them.

This point is extremely important: it is certainly not crazy to hope for the best, as long as you have back-up plans in case things don't turn out.

Fortunately, the human brain seems to be very good at doing both of those things simultaneously. We all seem to be adept at making plans for the worst eventualities and then enjoying and appreciating events if they turn out better.

Think, for example, of the effect of making your will. Nobody enjoys doing that, but most people get to it eventually, particularly once they have children. We all know that we will not be around to hear this document when it is read, yet the effect of making a will is neither paralyzing nor depressing. We don't sink into a trough of depression once it's done. In fact, it's almost the opposite: once we have planned for that eventuality, we can enjoy life more, rather than less.

That's proof that planning for the worst does not stop us from hoping for the best. Plans do not take away all hope.

Things We All Hope For

So hope is the expectation of a good outcome. And being an emotion, not a logical calculation, hope has nothing to do with statistics or math. You can hope to win the lottery when the odds are one in forty-five million. You can hope to win a coin-toss when the odds are one in two. You can hope for sunshine soon, even during a thunderstorm.

The statistics don't define the hope, because as we have seen, hope is the *feeling* we have when we think about a situation that is yet to be decided and anticipate a favorable outcome.

If that is what hope consists of, what are its components?

We all can, and do, hope for many different things, not just for one single thing. When we first hear a diagnosis of any medical condition, a cancer particularly, the first thing we all hope for is that it will be cured. Everyone hopes that the disease will be completely eliminated, never to return.

Now as I've emphasized from the very beginning of this book, that particular hope—of cure—can be achieved in about half of all cases. But even when cure *is* achieved, you may have to wait several years before you know *for certain* that the disease is not going to come back. During that time, before you *know* that the ending is happy, you *hope* for it.

Hope is the emotional bridge over the gulf between the present uncertainty and the future desired objective.

Hope of cure, however, of a perfect and certain happy ending, is not the only hope there is. Even if cure is not possible, there are still many appropriate and legitimate things that can be hoped for. And if you are told that cure is not guaranteed, or not *yet* guaranteed, that is not the same as taking away all hope. You can hear that news and still maintain hope.

Facing the facts is not the same as abandoning all hope.

I emphasize this point, because a lot of people (healthcare professionals as well as the general public) used to believe that it was somehow wrong to tell the truth to patients because truth (unless it was a pronouncement of cure) would take away their hope, and that was somehow wrong and harmful.

Nowadays, we have strong ethical, moral, practical, and even legal grounds for rejecting that view completely.

Even if cure is not (currently) a legitimate object of hope, there is a long list of things that are. Look at the items in the following list. My guess is that as you read the list you'll be saying to yourself, "Oh, of course, everybody hopes for *that*," or "Well, obviously, *that* stays on the wish list."

This list is the equivalent of Eric Cassell's timetable of flights, the list of Plan Bs that you have in your pocket as you run down the concourse.

We are all capable of hoping for the best even while we are preparing for the worst.

The Many Facets of Hope

Thing Hoped For	Achievable	
	Yes	No
Having a general understanding of the medical situation	✓	
Being able to ask some questions about what's going on	✓	
Good control of symptoms, including pain	✓	
Not being abandoned by your doctor and medical team	✓	
Keeping your friends	✓	
Help when you're feeling overwhelmed	✓	
Not putting people off when you're feeling low	✓	
Planning for family, kids, finances, etc.	✓	
Not being ruined financially	✓	
Having some input into the decisions	✓	

"Do I Always Have to Have a Positive Attitude?"

Cancer and the Mind

It is almost accepted as conventional wisdom that a strong will and determination have a major effect on the course of a cancer. So widely is it accepted, that what you are about to read in this section will probably cause considerable surprise.

The Simple Answer

There is a simple answer to the question, "Must I always have a positive attitude?" That simple, honest, and straightforward answer is, "No."

Even though the data are now very clear, this question for some reason is still widely thought of as "out there." The question of the effect of the mind on the cancer process seems to remain a big issue, and people still think of it as an undecided and open question.

But the data are clear: You will *not* do yourself any harm or make your disease any worse by having, as everybody does, moments of feeling low.

Attitude, Illness and History

There is a very long tradition of believing that attitude can affect the course of disease. It started at least two millennia ago with leprosy and continued in more modern times with tuberculosis, which was widely believed to be caused by having an artistic temperament and not eating properly. That same basic concept—that the patient's attitude or mind is responsible for the course (or even the cause) of the disease—continued with diseases such as syphilis, and then the cancers. Its most recent incarnation in the cancer field was the hypothesis put forward by Yale surgeon Bernie Siegel and, as you'll see, his hypothesis was actually disproved by his own studies.

It's difficult to be clear headed about an issue as emotionally loaded as cancer and the mind, but I think that going through the background and the data in a steady systematic way is helpful.

Coping with the Unintelligible

Step back for a moment and think about how the human species copes with things that seem to be arbitrary and unintelligible.

The bottom line is this: whenever we see something we don't understand, we tend to ascribe a hidden cause to it. It is a characteristic human trait which we have always exhibited in our behavior when facing the unknown. It is true, for example, of natural disasters and catastrophes such as earthquakes and floods and even thunderstorms, all of which were originally thought by our ancestors to be caused by the vengeance or anger of the gods.

The same trait of human behavior is seen in our attitudes to illness. We have a strong tendency to deal with the sense of disquiet and unease caused by a feeling of, "I don't know what caused this" by seeking the slightly more comforting, "It must be due to something."

We've done it for centuries. Long before Robert Koch discovered the bacterium that causes tuberculosis, there was a common popular opinion that people with tuberculosis brought it on themselves by being of an artistic temperament or of delicate sensibilities: the stereotype was the artist starving in a garret.

There was even a word for it. Tuberculosis used to be called *phthisis*, and the type of personality thought to be artistic, delicate, and sensitive was called the *phthisical personality*. If an artist developed tuberculosis, he was the cause of his own undoing, or so the common wisdom had it.

Sure enough, many very famous artists did starve in garrets and several died of tuberculosis, but there was no link between these two facts. Very few people noticed that the artist starving in a garret might have a relative or friend in the same room who was coughing all night and in the process was coughing what we now know as *tubercle bacilli* all over the artist. Once the antituberculous antibiotics were discovered in the 1940s, the treatment of tuberculosis changed dramatically and the entire myth of the phthisical personality disappeared.

Before the modern era, ulcerative colitis was thought to be caused by an obsessive personality, schizophrenia by a dysfunctional family, and Down's syndrome, a chromosomal abnormality, by the parents being intoxicated at the moment of conception!

That's what's going on now with the cancers. It involves two types of widely held beliefs: first, that an attitude of mind can *cause* a cancer to develop and, second, that a positive attitude of mind has a big influence on the *course* of a cancer.

I'm going to deal with these two beliefs separately.

"Did My Mind or My Attitude Cause My Cancer?"

First, we have to accept the fact that most cancers appear without an obvious cause or precipitating event.

There are, of course, the smoking-related cancers (although even with those, lawyers in the United States have managed to prolong the debate and create the impression that there is some doubt about causality). But apart from those cancers, in the great majority of cases, there is no immediately obvious and intuitively satisfactory explanation for why (or when) a cancer makes it presence felt.

Seen from a distance, then, most cancers appear to be arbitrary and unintelligible events. And as I've just pointed out, our tendency as human beings is to cope with the threat posed by an arbitrary event by trying to ascribe causes to it which make it more intelligible.

Healers, doctors, writers, patients, and people from every discipline and every part of our society suggest—some even state as a proven fact—that by some means cancer is the outward expression of unresolved emotional processes, involving either mood or life events (or both). There are many variations on this theme, but in general, it suggests that the person who later develops cancer has partly contributed to causing it by bottling up emotions, by not expressing anger, by allowing external stresses to build up internally or by some other psychological process.

"Why Do So Many People Believe You Cause Your Own Cancer?"

The motive—or urge—that underlies this belief is easy to see.

If it were proven to be true, that cancers were caused by a bad attitude, then the world would be a more understandable place, and perhaps more fair and just. It would, in some respects, be a form of justice if the people who held unhealthy attitudes (not related to any of their actions such as smoking) had a high risk of developing cancer, and if the people who had the correct attitudes or beliefs could thereby reduce the chances of getting the disease.

There are many factors that make it easy to believe this. And I think it's worth spending a moment or two discussing the various strings to this bow, because the bombardment of (apparent) information is so intense and unrelenting that most people feel, "I've heard it so often and from so many different sources that it must be true."

But it isn't. When it comes to this particular bit of conventional wisdom, billions of people can be wrong!

"That Makes Sense": The Power of Individual Stories

Almost everybody knows someone, or knows *of* someone, who was diagnosed with a cancer shortly after a time of great stress.

A man's wife dies and three months later he is found to have cancer of the bowel. A woman nurses her dying mother through the last year of her life, and shortly afterwards finds a lump in her breast that turns out to be malignant. Another woman looking after her daughter on her own endures three years of high stress and anxiety while her daughter deals with her drug addiction. Shortly after things begin to settle down, the mother is found to have a cancer. An important lawyer in a law firm is suddenly "let go" after fifteen years. Following six months of deep depression and feelings of uselessness, he is diagnosed with cancer of the lung.

There are lots of stories such as these, and they all make intuitive sense. It seems logical that a catastrophic stress—a divorce, a bereavement, a dismissal—should be followed by a catastrophic illness such as cancer. Yet, although it seems logical and makes intuitive sense, it may not be true. Several factors may contribute to the intuitive credibility of this idea:

Set Thinking

The phrase *set thinking* describes the pattern that we all have of putting things we see into groups, in other words filing our experience in sets of data. (It has nothing to do with set meaning fixed or unalterable, as in *set in his ways*.)

If you have just bought a blue Volkswagen, let's say, then every time you see another blue Volkswagen, you will notice it. It will have some special significance. Probably you never much noticed blue

Volkswagens before. As a result, after you have bought your blue Volkswagen, it will seem to you that there is a sudden surge in popularity of blue Volkswagens. That might be true. Maybe you have started a fashion trend! It is much more likely, however, that the number of blue Volkswagens on the road has not altered. It is just that you are now noticing the ones that are there.

The same is true of individual stories that we hear about people who have had a cancer. We make a mental note only of the events that seem linked in a way that makes sense to us: the divorce, the bereavement, the dismissal and so on. But we don't notice those stories of people who have divorces, bereavement, or dismissal and who *don't* develop a cancer. Nor do we note those people who have been diagnosed with a cancer who have *not* had a trauma.

In other words, there is a particular set of stories—where cancer follows trauma—that we remember and take note of. We do not know whether people who have divorces have more cancer than people who do not, nor whether people who have cancer are more likely to have been recently divorced or not.

Furthermore, there are factors that we do know are important in the causation of cancer, but which may not be obvious in the story that we hear. For example, the lawyer who was dismissed might have been a heavy smoker for many years, although he might well have given up smoking five years ago. If that were the case, then his lung cancer might be explained more easily by the cigarettes than the dismissal.

So we need to know whether a group of people who have, let us say, gone through major stress in the last two years have an increased chance of getting a cancer, compared to another group of the same age who have not had significant life events.

In fact, a recent example does exactly that, and it's so important that I want to discuss it in some detail.

Stress and the Recurrence of Cancers: Some Facts

Despite the general view that this issue is still undecided and open, there are many studies which have been done in which the verdict is clear.

At the risk of seeming to be a bit pedantic, I'll mention a few of them.

In 1989, cancer researchers at a major center in the United Kingdom studied a group of fifty women and asked them how stressful their lives had been. They then compared those fifty women to a control group and found that when there was severe stress in the woman's life, the chance of the breast cancer recurring was several times higher.

This was an extremely important finding. If it was true, if stress in your life allows the cancer to recur more easily, then it would strongly suggest that reducing the stress in a woman's life may reduce the chance of her breast cancer recurring.

The researchers then planned a second study which would address that suggestion.

The first study had a real design flaw. The investigators had asked women to assess their stress levels at the time of recurrence, and it was quite possible that the turmoil of the recurrence might increase their own assessment of their stress level. If that were so, then a retrospective study might show a correlation that wasn't really there.

In the second study, the researchers asked the women to assess the stress level before recurrence.

They followed a group of women between 1991 and 1998, and the published their results in 2002. The study showed that there was *no correlation between stress and the recurrence of breast cancer.*

In other words, these researchers had done a valuable and reliable thing. They had come across something which might have been important. They set up a second study to see whether or not it was. And their second study, scrupulously conducted on a flawless design, showed that there was not a genuine effect after all. Stress does not increase the chance of breast cancer recurring.

The set thinking which triggered the researchers' interest, and everybody else's, was exactly that. It was not an indicator of some mysterious relationship between stress and breast cancer.

There are many other studies which all support the same point. Studies of large groups of people have now been done in an attempt to prove or disprove the idea that either the mood of the person or the events that happen in a person's life may contribute to the cause of cancer. At present, these do not show that there is a causal relationship.

Depression
There is no confirmed evidence that depression contributes to the cause of cancer. One major study (*Journal of the American Medical Association*, 1990) evaluated communities in five cities and compared the incidence of cancer after a period of ten years. If depression was even a minor contributory cause to cancer, the study had a very high chance of showing that connection. In fact, there was no link, and the people with depression had the same chance of developing cancer as the general population.

In terms of psychological stress, it has long been known that bereavement is one of the most stressful. A study in Israel looked for an increase in cancer among parents who had lost a child. No such increase in cancer was found.

Taking all these pieces of evidence together, I think that we can be confident that there is a genuine verdict.

The Verdict: Stress Doesn't Cause Cancers
There is no credible evidence whatever that stress itself, as opposed to a behavior such as smoking cigarettes, contributes to the cause of any cancers, or even affects the course of a cancer. To put it simply, this belief is part of blaming the patient, a traditional public way of dealing

with all manner of diseases until they were understood. Stress may well be unpleasant, and it may affect all manner of things including our relationships to other people and our ability to drive a car or make decisions. But it has never been, and it is not now, a contributory factor in the causes of cancer.

"Can My Mind Change the Outcome?"

So stress and mood, by themselves, do not cause cancers.

But it is also widely believed that, once you have a cancer, a positive attitude and a good mental state positively will affect the outcome of the disease.

That idea is intellectually appealing: it implies that you can make a difference. But is it true?

Actually there are many studies in this difficult area, and they are quoted often and widely, and often wrongly!

In 1979, a study by two London researchers (Drs. Greer and Morris) interested in the psychological aspects of cancer showed some very remarkable findings.

Their study involved a group of patients with diagnosed breast cancer. With semi-structured interviews the doctors assessed the attitudes that the patients had to their illness before the diagnosis was made. They then correlated those attitudes to their survival. Extraordinarily, they found that patients who were extremely angry and patients who went into denial did very well. By contrast, patients who simply coped with the disease and carried on as best they could, and patients who went into a helpless and hopeless state did less well.

This paper was very significant, and the *methodology* of classifying patients' reaction in this particular way has been used in many centers since. However, the *results* have never been successfully repeated in another study. This is somewhat unexpected, since the original study was on a small group of patients and should not be difficult to repeat. But this 1979 study remains a single interesting observation.

The Bristol Cancer Help Centre is one of Britain's most well-known complementary medicine centers for cancer patients and the treatment there includes a wide range of psychological and spiritual techniques as well as a stringent diet.

In their early publications, the Centre had claimed that its treatments could and would prolong life and it later collaborated with conventional physicians in a study of people with advanced breast cancer. Patients at the Bristol were matched with approximately twice that number of patients at conventional centers.

The results showed that the chance of dying was actually higher at the Bristol Centre than in the conventional centers. The publication of this paper caused immense political furor.

Nevertheless, the data did not show that patients lived longer at the Bristol Centre. And the conclusions in the paper bear comparison with a similar study (*New England Journal of Medicine*, 1991) which compared patients at a complementary medicine clinic in the United States with patients in a conventional center. The same conclusion is supported by the two Siegel studies described below.

Dr. Bernie Siegel is a Yale-trained surgeon who specialized in cancer and in recent years has concentrated on the psychological aspects of serious illness, particularly cancer. In the late 1980s he suggested that a positive attitude could change the course of cancers, and he started an immense public debate and discussion, with literally millions of people supporting his view.

This is old news. But it's worth looking at because I think that it will all happen again. I suspect that there will new books and new theories suggesting that patients can make their cancer resolve (or at least stabilize) if they try hard enough and want to enough. As I have already hinted (and as I recap at the end of this section) I think there is a critically important issue underlying this.

Bernie Siegel (he likes to be called "Bernie" not "Dr. Siegel") noticed that in some patients certain psychological characteristics and behavior patterns seemed to be associated with a longer survival. He called these patients *exceptional cancer patients* or E-CaPs. He started therapy groups and meetings of E-CaPs and of those who wanted to be E-CaPs.

He published several popular books about the influence of the mind on serious diseases, particularly cancer. In his books, through stories and examples, Bernie implied that psychological attitudes were a determinant of survival. In other words, he implied that the state of mind of the patient affected the progress of the cancer.

He then collaborated in two studies, the first a pilot study with small numbers, the second a larger study. Both of these studies showed that being an E-Cap did not prolong survival. In other words, Bernie's own studies tested his hypothesis and disproved it.

As I said to Bernie at the time, when I interviewed him for a television series, his participation in this kind of research is admirable. That sort of intellectual honesty and curiosity sets him apart from the majority of other popular figures in this field. It is to his lasting credit that he carefully and deliberately set out to test the idea that E-CaPs do better than other cancer patients. The fact that there was no demonstrable benefit in terms of *longer life* does not diminish the value that the groups have for the people who attend. But it does support the conclusion that E-CaP groups do not extend life.

By contrast, Dr. David Spiegel is a psychiatrist practicing in a university hospital in Stanford, California. In the late 1970s and early 1980s, Dr. Spiegel had set up some psychotherapy support groups for women with breast cancer. These group sessions were carefully designed and did not simply encourage the participants to take a positive attitude or hope that things would turn out better if they did. In fact, the groups did several things that were unusual. First, the participants in the groups were actively encouraged to face the facts of their situation, and to confront—and cope with—the possibility of dying of breast cancer. Second, the groups actively encouraged networking and social contacts between the participants outside the group sessions. This original research study was designed to see if sessions like this could improve the quality of life. The results clearly showed that these techniques *did* improve the quality of life.

After several years had elapsed, and Bernie Siegel's concept of hope as a therapeutic agent became popular, Dr. Spiegel decided to see if the group sessions had made any difference to survival, fully expecting that there would be no effect. To his surprise the long-term follow-up of the women who had attended these groups showed that they lived longer than the people who had not.

This was a very important finding because it was the first, and the only, piece of evidence derived from a prospective study that shows that survival might be affected by psychological and social factors.

I met and interviewed Dr. Spiegel as part of the same television series and found him to be a serious, thoughtful, and original researcher. Perhaps the most important aspect of his work is that his immediate response to his 1989 findings was to insist that the work be repeated in several different cities to see if his results were valid and reproducible.

That process, appropriately, took many years. When eventually the research data were analyzed, it was found that there was no effect. Attending therapy groups, beneficial though it is for the quality of life, did not prolong survival or affect the course of breast cancer in any way.

This probably means one of two things. Either the 1989 results were a chance finding; for instance, there was some difference in the two groups that we were not aware of, some aspect of the tumors perhaps.

Or there was some factor at work in Stanford in 1989 which cannot be reproduced or translated to other centers.

Dr. Spiegel also had many interesting views on the meaning of his research, and of the clear and palpable value of support in coping with a cancer and treatment.

As he said, think of a single person walking through Central Park at two in the morning alone. Then think of the same person doing the same thing in a group of twenty people. The effect of company, of community, of support from your friends and relatives, is enormous. Feeling alone and isolated is a terrible feeling in itself, and a circle of supportive and confiding friends make it much easier for you to cope with almost anything.

The Bottom Line: Blaming the Patient

As I have said above, there is a long history of humankind blaming the patient, and it is possible that contemporary attitudes about the mind and cancer are simply part of that long tradition. Of course, there are some cancers where a patient's *actions* are a known contributing factor—smoking in cancers of the lung, mouth, bladder, and pancreas, for example, and sunlight in skin cancers. But most of the other cancers arrive mysteriously, and apparently randomly.

We do not like that randomness, so we impose an orderly structure on the events, whether it exists or not.

In the case of the cancers: we blame the patient.

Yes, it is remotely possible that the mind *does* play an important role and the patient *is* in part to blame. But it does not look like that so far.

I suspect that much of this feeling that cancer is caused by the patient in some way is humankind's time-honored way of dealing with the discomfort of the unknown.

Blaming the patient helps people who do not have the disease feel safe, and perhaps superior. If we can identify something the patient has done, and has *chosen* to do, that caused the cancer, then maybe, the reasoning goes, *we* will not get that cancer if we are careful. Hence our desire to find things in patients' lives that set them apart from healthy people. I think it is likely many of the examples from the past illustrate this basic trait of human behavior.

It may make us feel better at the expense of the patient, but it simply isn't a reflection of the truth.

"What Can I Do to Help Myself?"

Gaining More Control

In coping with an uncertain and potentially serious condition, everybody needs two things: an accurate understanding of the situation to reduce the sense of fear and helplessness; and a feeling of community, of not being alone, to reduce the sense of isolation and loneliness. I hope that this book will provide both of those things for the cancer patient and the family, and give a real sense of purpose and meaning.

You've Already Started

One more time for good measure: the word *cancer* is probably the scariest word in the English language. The word itself almost always brings with it deep-seated feelings of dread and fear, and those feelings often cause a sensation of helplessness, of being almost paralyzed and powerless, and of not having any control over events.

Many of those feelings come from thinking of all of the different cancers as one single terrible disease. I very much hope that this book has done something to change that way of thinking and of feeling. Obtaining a clear understanding of your own particular situation—

your particular cancer, the stage, the treatment plan, and so on—is the most important way to cope with the fear that so often lurks in the background.

That's what I've been trying to do through this whole book. And I hope that in that process you've regained some of your balance, some feeling of control, and some sense of direction.

The "You Are Here" Sticker

Getting your sense of direction back is a major part of regaining your balance, and what you need for that is an overview, a general picture—a map of the forest, not just a catalog of the trees. Very often you need to get that kind of map from books like this one, because your own medical team doesn't have the time to explain that big picture.

I hope this book has done that for you, and that it has given you a map of what was previously unknown territory, with a prominent "You Are Here" sticker to give you some sense of where you are and where the various paths and options go.

Feeling bewildered and lost also isolates you from your friends and relatives. If you don't really know how you're doing, it can become very difficult for you to talk to your friends. They ask you questions, because they want to know and to help. And if you can't answer, you might be tempted not to continue the conversation. Some people (and doctors are often among them when it's their turn to be patients!) even feel a touch guilty about not understanding what's happening with their own medical condition. They have a feeling that they ought to know or even that everybody else understands the situation and they don't. These types of feelings are made even worse in the atmosphere of a busy clinic where everyone is working at maximum efficiency and everybody seems to know precisely that they are doing. You need to know where on that map the "You Are Here" sticker is situated at any given moment.

Once you have that general idea, you'll find it easier to get support from the people around you, which is probably one of the most important factors in affecting the quality of your everyday living.

Friends

The real sense of community—of friendship, of genuine contact—in a conversation comes when both parties are able to let down their own defenses enough to talk about what they actually feel. That's why the sections in this book on communication are so useful. If you can name and acknowledge the deep feelings that you have—fear, sadness, embarrassment, guilt, anger, frustration, disappointment—you are doing an incredibly important thing. You are making real contact: you and the other person are being real friends. And some of us think that real friendship is the only thing that counts. Those moments of deep contact are truly memorable, last forever, and unlike almost everything else in our daily lives don't fade, go out of fashion, or wrinkle!

Support Groups

You may also want to think about joining a support group. This is a very personal choice. Some people gain real comfort and support from the experience of other people and from hearing their stories and practical suggestions and tips. (Some of these tips are news, and useful, to doctors when we hear about them!) Other people just don't like the feeling of a group. I suggest that you give it a try. The atmosphere is each group is very individual, and often friendships are created that are of great value and long duration. Many people who don't think of themselves as support-group types are actually pleasantly surprised when they try it. It doesn't feel the way they thought it would, the support is palpable, and the fears of confrontation or embarrassment turn out to be groundless. So ask at your clinic about support groups in your area, think about it, and perhaps give it a try. You may be very surprised.

The Net

Then there is the Internet. The number of sites that you get if you search for the word *cancer* is probably above three million.

There are two secrets to using the Net if you want to avoid giving yourself panic attacks or anxiety: first, know the kind of questions you want to ask and, second, remember that you are trying to acquire *general* information, not to become an expert in your own condition. There's nothing intrinsically wrong with doing exhaustive searches and reading about dozens of different studies and treatments and claims, but it may make you even more distressed and anxious. It is probably better to go to a few trustworthy Web sites set up by major cancer centers, hospitals, or cancer charities and support organizations.

The problem with the Internet is that anyone can say anything on it. There may be a Web site which states, with what seems like learned authority, that all cancers can be cured by a diet of grapefruit skins and coconut, or by breathing in a different way, or wearing magnets or ampoules of electrically-charged fluid.

Quite often, wide-ranging grand claims like that are put out by a single person or a small group of people who have their hearts in the right place but who know nothing about the cancers, and have no contact with any cancer researchers or treatment centers. Actually, a fair amount of the "wilder" Internet information about the cancers is like that, right-hearted but unsupported by fact or experiment: wishful thinking and speculation disguised as fact. Your problem is that you can't necessarily detect that from the first visit to the Web site.

To help you, we've listed some of the real and trustworthy Web sites. In Appendix B on page 269 you'll find a list of Web sites that we can personally vouch for. They represent not only the current treatment approaches but also ongoing research (and some of the research studies that are in progress as well). Visit one of these sites first. It will help you find your feet and be less swayed by the more outlandish claims, however optimistic and enticing they may seem.

"Will There Ever Be a Cure for Cancer?"'

The question, "Will there ever be a cure for a cancer?" must be the most common question that any cancer physician or researcher is asked.

For at least eight decades there has been a general feeling that the cure for cancer is just around the corner. This view of the situation (and this is my own opinion) has been promoted by both the general public, who want to see the end of what they regard as a single dreadful disease, and by the medical profession who genuinely want to be the people who do it. Since the early twentieth century, the press (and later the electronic media) made a very big deal of this, and have hailed any advance in cancer research or cancer treatment as an imminent cure.

Only recently have we all become much more temperate in our attitudes. In the last few years it has become more common for oncologists to be quoted as saying things like, "We need to do more testing, but this treatment might be useful for a number of patients with breast cancer that develops after the menopause." Researchers are nowadays less likely to be prompted into saying that their work is a major breakthrough, but are more likely to say that it opens up new avenues of research, or that the drug is clearly active in treating cancers in mice, but we don't yet know if it has similar actions or any actions in humans.

In other words, just as there is no single disease called *cancer*, there will not be a single cure for all the cancers. What we will see in the future is what we are seeing now: small or moderate advances in one or several of the cancers, but not all. Unfortunately it is an illusion that there will be a single substance which, when discovered or invented, has the power of reversing the cancer process in all the two hundred or more cancers. It is something that everybody, patients and professionals alike, would dearly like to see, but there will not be one single substance that is "the cure."

Instead there will be steady advances in reversing the cancer in some types, controlling it in others, and improving treatment by increasing the activity of the medications while decreasing their side effects. It will be, as it has been for the last fifty years, a large number of small advances that stimulate new researches and new discoveries.

There is tremendous hope—hope of controlling the disease, and of coping with it more easily and for a longer time if it cannot be cured—but just as there are so many different cancers, so there are so many different treatments and treatment approaches.

We are generally doing fairly well, and "the search for the single cure" is an unreal yardstick by which we fail to appreciate the progress we are actually making.

You Are Not Alone

I hope that this book really has given you a firm overview and navigational guide—a broad map of the territory. Most of all, I hope that it has helped you get your balance back and has helped you realize that the cancers are a group of diseases, all of which have different implications and different treatment options from each other.

Even more important, the cancers—like the vast majority of diseases—are medical conditions that we should all be able to discuss openly, without fear or embarrassment or dread.

The overtones and connotations attached to the single word *cancer* have for many decades now made everyone talk in whispers or keep totally silent. That atmosphere of hushed foreboding always made rational and helpful conversation difficult or even impossible.

But times are changing, as they should. Because when you come right down to it, the word *cancer* is exactly that—a word, not a sentence.

Tables

Table 1. The Features of a Cancer that the Pathologist Assesses

Table 1 and Table 2 contain a general and approximate guide to the (literally) hundreds of features that pathologists assess. This is an oversimplification of course, but it will give you some idea of how the appearance of the cancer under the microscope can predict how the cancer is going to behave, and also why the pathologist's report is a very important factor in planning treatment.

Feature	What the Pathologist Assesses	What This Can Mean
The Grade of the Tumor (= How Aggressive It Appears to Be)		
Size	It may seem obvious, but in some tumors the size of the cancer makes a difference, and smaller cancers behave differently from larger ones. In many cancers, the exact size is part of the assessment of the primary cancer and is an important factor to be taken into account.	
Type of tumor	There are many subtypes in this feature: whether the cancer is forming glands, makes mucus, contains clear (serous) fluid; whether the cells are small (very important in lung cancers and in lymphomas), or flat cells like skin cells (squamous).	Sometimes (but not always) the subtype of the cancer has an influence on the way it behaves, and sometimes the subtype helps predict how the cancer should be treated (e.g., response to chemotherapy).

Feature	What the Pathologist Assesses	What This Can Mean
The Grade of the Tumor (= How Aggressive It Appears to Be)		
Tissue of origin: where does it come from (e.g., breast, lung, bowel, etc.)?	This is a crucial point—and in many cases the origin is immediately apparent. Sometimes, particularly if the cells are very undifferentiated or if there has been a lot of damage to the biopsy specimen, it may be difficult to say in which tissue it began. This is particularly true when examining secondary tumors, say, in a lymph node or lung biopsy.	The tissue of origin is extremely important. If breast cancer spreads to the lung, say, then it still behaves like breast cancer (not like lung cancer) and is likely to respond to drugs used in breast cancer. If it is lung cancer that has spread to the bone, or the liver, then it behaves like lung cancer. Hence the pathologist's opinion as to where the cancer originated is of great importance.
Differentiation: how close is the resemblance of the cancer cells to normal cells of that tissue?	How many features of the original normal cells are still there in the cancer cells? If most of them are there, the tumor is *well differentiated* or *low grade*. If very few, the cancer is *poorly differentiated* or *high grade*.	Low-grade tumors usually grow more slowly and have a lower tendency to spread. High-grade tumors are usually more aggressive in their behavior, and usually have a greater tendency to spread to distant parts of the body.
Features inside the cancer cells: nucleus, and nuclear/ cytoplasm ratio	Very large nuclei inside the cells—particularly if there is little cytoplasm (the jelly that fills the rest of the cell)—suggest aggressive behavior. In some tumors there may be several nuclei per cell and this is also a sign of aggression.	These features are almost universal in all cancers— the smaller and the more normal-looking the nuclei, the better.

Feature	What the Pathologist Assesses	What This Can Mean
The Grade of the Tumor (= How Aggressive It Appears to Be)		
Mitotic figures: how many cells are actively dividing at the moment?	When a cell divides, the process (mitosis) makes a visible change in the cell's appearance. If lots of cells are doing this at any one time, it suggests that the tumor is rapidly growing.	The smaller the number of mitotic figures that are seen the better—a very useful guide in some tumors, particularly sarcomas and ovarian tumors.
Architecture (gland formation, etc.)	Normal tissues have a characteristic pattern of the way the cells are arranged (glands and ducts in breast tissue, glands and finger-like processes in bowel tissue, etc.). The degree to which these features are kept (or lost) also indicates the degree of aggressive behavior.	The more that the "normal architecture" is preserved in a cancer the better.
Invading Into Surrounding Areas & Nodes		
Depth of invasion	In many tissues, how deep the tumor penetrates is important (for example in uterine cancer and in melanoma).	Depth of invasion can make a big difference to the staging and the whole treatment approach (uterine cancer, vulva cancer and melanomas are examples).
The basement membrane	Many tissues (bowel, for example) have a very clear boundary between the top layers and the bottom layers. This is the basement membrane, and how much and in what manner the cancer goes through it is often important.	Whether or not the cancer goes through the basement membrane may affect the staging of the cancer (in bowel, for example) and how the treatment is planned.

Feature	What the Pathologist Assesses	What This Can Mean
Lymph nodes	Lymph nodes are the local filtering stations: in most cancers (but not all) they are the first sites for spread. In many tumors, the amount of cancer invasion is also an important feature.	In most cases, whether or not the cancer has spread to the nearby lymph nodes is a major factor in deciding how aggressive it is likely to be.
Vascular invasion	In many cases, the pathologist can see if the cancer cells are invading into the small blood vessels or capillaries or small lymph vessels in the neighborhood.	In some cancers—breast, particularly—invasion into lymph vessels or capillaries is a very important feature, and suggests a risk of spread even if the cancer hasn't actually spread to nearby lymph nodes.
Margins: has all the cancer in that area been removed by the surgery—are the margins of the surgical specimen or biopsy clear of cancer?	Sometimes a cancer can spread in a way that is not easy for the surgeon to see simply by visual inspection. If the cancer is present right at the borders of the surgically removed specimen, then further surgery may be required.	If there are *positive margins*, this is may require more surgery or additional local treatment such as radiotherapy, depending on the tumor and the local situation.

Table 2. Special Stains that Can Be Done on Some Cancers

Using special stains, the pathologist can find out whether the cancer cells have certain molecules on the surface, and that may tell something about the type or subtype of cell.		
Receptors	Receptors are complex molecules that bind with (receive) hormones or other messenger-molecules. They may be on the cell surface or in the cytoplasm, as is the case with estrogen receptors and progesterone receptors.	In the case of breast cancer, if estrogen receptors are present, then hormone medications such as tamoxifen have a high chance of being effective. If the receptors are not present, then hormone therapies will not work.
Other molecular targets: EGF, VEGF, etc.	When certain molecular groups are found on the surface of the cancer cells, it may indicate behavior that is different from the average and/or whether particular biologic agents are likely to be effective.	Receptors may predict something about the cancer cells in themselves (for example, the *her2/neu* receptor on breast cancer usually denotes faster growth) or sensitivity to an agent (estrogen receptors mean that cancer has a high chance of responding to hormone medications, *her2/neu* receptors mean that the drug Herceptin has a good chance of producing a response).
Some Other Markers Often Used		
Mucin stains	When there is mucin-production in the cancer, it indicates certain types of bowel and stomach cancers, and among ovarian cancers a particular subtype.	

Cytokeratin-7 cytokeratin-20	An example of a molecular marker often found on colon and on ovarian cancer cells.	
CEA	A molecular marker found in many colon cancer cells and many breast cancer cells.	
Calretinin	Commonly found on a rare cancer, mesothelioma.	
Melan-A	A marker found only in melanoma cancers.	

Table 3. The Most Common Types of Tests and What They Mean

Test	How It Works	What It's Like	How It Helps
1. Blood Tests			
A. Blood Tests That Assess Whether or Not a Tissue or Organ Is Working Well			
Blood Count (includes hemoglobin, white cells & platelets)	The standard blood count (CBC) is the routine test done most frequently. The result is usually available promptly.	Test done on sample of blood.	Blood components are produced in the bone marrow: if there is no clear reason for abnormalities, a bone marrow sample may sometimes be needed.
Hemoglobin (Hb)	The hemoglobin is the red pigment that carries oxygen.	Test done on sample of blood.	If the hemoglobin is low (anemia) you many feel tired or short of breath. Sometimes a transfusion is required.

Test	How It Works	What It's Like	How It Helps
1. Blood Tests			
A. Blood Tests That Assess Whether or Not a Tissue or Organ Is Working Well			
White Cells (WBC)	The total white cell count and particularly the type of white cells called the *neutrophils* are important in deciding whether chemotherapy can be given.	Test done on sample of blood.	If the white cells (particularly the neutrophils) are low, you may be susceptible to infection and fever, requiring treatment with antibiotics. Delay of chemotherapy or use of biologics such as Neupogen to increase the white cell count may be considered.
Platelets	The platelets are small components of the blood that are major factors in forming blood clots.	Test done on sample of blood.	If the platelets are low (thrombocytopenia) you may be susceptible to bruises or bleeding (e.g., gum or rectal bleeding).
Creatinine	A compound produced by the body's metabolism and excreted by the kidneys.	Test done on sample of blood.	If the creatinine level is high, it may mean that the kidneys are not working normally or there is dehydration.

Test	How It Works	What It's Like	How It Helps
1. Blood Tests			
A. Blood Tests That Assess Whether or Not a Tissue or Organ Is Working Well			
Electrolytes ("Lytes")	Sodium, potassium, and chloride levels in the blood are upset in many abnormalities of fluid and kidney control.	Test done on sample of blood.	Unexpected abnormalities may indicate many different underlying problems, and a wide range of treatment approaches.
Liver Function Tests (LFTs)	Three enzymes called *transaminases* and one called *alkaline phosphatase* become elevated if the liver is abnormal.	Test done on sample of blood.	The transaminases become elevated if the liver cells are inflamed, and the alkaline phosphatase rises if part of the bile duct system is blocked.
Clotting Screen	A group of tests done to assess whether the blood can clot normally. Includes a test called *Prothrombin Time* (PT) and a comparison of this to normal levels the INR.	Test done on sample of blood.	Used to assess the effect of blood thinners and detect other abnormalities in the clotting system.
Albumin	Main component of the protein in your blood, produced by the liver.	Test done on sample of blood.	Can be low in any illness that goes on for a long time. Useful guide to your nutritional status.

Test	How It Works	What It's Like	How It Helps
1. Blood Tests			
B. Tumor Markers: Blood Tests That Assess the Amount of Tumor			
CEA	Carcino-Embryonic Antigen is a protein produced by some cancer cells (particularly breast, colo-rectal and some lung cancers).	Test done on sample of blood.	If abnormal the CEA is a useful test to monitor the effect of treatment on the cancer.
CA.125	A protein produced by cancer of the ovary cells (and occasionally by noncancerous problems in the abdomen).	Test done on sample of blood.	If abnormal the CA.125 is a useful test to monitor the effect of treatment on the cancer.
PSA	Prostate Specific Antigen is produced by prostate cells and doesn't leak out into the blood unless the covering of the prostate gland is damaged (usually by cancer, sometimes by inflammation).	Test done on sample of blood.	If abnormal when there is known and diagnosed cancer of the prostate, the PSA level is a very useful test for monitoring the effect of treatment on the cancer.

Test	How It Works	What It's Like	How It Helps
B. Tumor Markers: Blood Tests That Assess the Amount of Tumor			
HCG	A hormone produced by testicular cancer and cancer of the placenta and a few others.	Test done on sample of blood.	Levels are reliable markers for monitoring treatment of the cancer, and are also early indications of recurrence.
AFP	A protein produced by testicular cancer and liver cancer cells.	Test done on sample of blood.	Levels are reliable markers for monitoring treatment of the cancer, and are also early indications of recurrence.
2. X-rays & Scans			
Chest X-ray	Shows lungs, size of heart, ribs and (to some extent) spine.	Usually taken with you standing up (straight on, and then sideways).	Many different abnormalities of the lung or of fluid outside the lungs (pleural effusion), enlargement of the heart or fluid around the heart, abnormalities in the ribs, and sometimes in the spine.

Test	How It Works	What It's Like	How It Helps
2. X-rays & Scans			
Bone X-rays	X-rays in bone tissue can show fractures of course, and areas of cancer if the cancer is either dissolving the bone (lytic) or making excess bone (sclerotic). X-rays are important in trying to decide if there is a risk of fracture.	X-rays of painful bones can be uncomfortable: positioning the arm or leg can sometimes be a trial. But usually it's only for a short while.	If the lesions are moderately big they can be seen on X-ray. Fractures can be seen as well.
Bone Scan	An injection of a small dose of the harmless isotope *technetium* is given, and then scans of your body are done with a special camera that detects where the technetium has gone.	You get a small intravenous injection, and then you have to lie down on a table while the gamma camera moves down the length of your body (on a gantry a few feet up).	Reliable indicator of metastases in some cancers (e.g., breast) but not all.

Test	How It Works	What It's Like	How It Helps
2. X-rays & Scans			
Ultrasound	Uses very high-frequency sound waves to examine internal organs.	You lie down while a microphone-like probe is passed over your abdomen (or into the vagina in assessing certain pelvic conditions).	Very useful in detecting abnormities inside the liver, the lymph nodes in the abdomen, the uterus and ovaries, and many other structures in the abdomen or pelvis (not so good at detecting small abnormalities inside the colon).
CT	Uses very sophisticated computer analysis of "slices" of X-rays taken up and down the body.	You lie on a moveable shelf which slides through a big doughnut-shaped machine. Totally painless!	A standard way of assessing many parts of the body.
MRI	Detects changes in the magnetic fields in your body after short surges of magnetic fields are applied. It so happens that this is very good at detecting water-containing tissues and is particularly effective in the brain and spinal cord.	Painless but claustrophobic! You lie down inside a plastic box while the magnetic field generator gives pulses which you do not feel! The machine is very noisy and it takes a half-hour or so, but it doesn't hurt at all.	Sometimes important when CT scans are not so useful (e.g., brain and spinal cord, and some other situations).

Test	How It Works	What It's Like	How It Helps
2. X-rays & Scans			
Gallium Scan	*Gallium* is an isotope which happens to be taken up by certain cells in the lymphoid group— so it's very good for Hodgkin's disease, some lymphomas and some other conditions.	It's just like a bone scan, but the injection is a different material.	Can be helpful in assessing the size and position of any tumor of Hodgkin's or certain lymphomas.
Mammograms	X-rays of the breast tissue.	Almost always reported as uncomfortable! The breast tissue needs to be compressed between glass plates to be X-rayed properly.	Mammograms may be abnormal in many benign conditions, and occasionally some cancers are not visible to X-rays.
PET Scans	(Not routine) Scan records a particular kind of electrical signal.	Very similar to a bone scan from your point of view.	Can be very useful in conjunction with CT scan results to image tumors.
Barium Enema	X-rays done after the colon has been filled with liquid that shows up on X-rays.	Uncomfortable. Liquid is passed by thin tube into the colon, then X-rays taken with you lying on your back and sides.	

Test	How It Works	What It's Like	How It Helps
3. Tests Used to Look Directly at a Tumor or Organ			
Colonoscopy	Long flexible tube is passed from the anus through all the length of the colon.	You will be heavily sedated so the procedure is usually not even uncomfortable. You have to drink a large amount of special fluid the night before.	Routine test (also used in screening) for tumors (cancers and polyps) of colon and rectum.
Bronchoscopy	Short flexible tube is passed down the trachea into the upper parts of the lungs.	Usually under heavy sedation or general anesthetic.	One method of assessing cancers of lung and airways.
Laryngoscopy	Short flexible tube is passed to the back of the throat to examine the larynx and the back of the nasal passages.	Mouth and throat are sprayed with local anesthetic. Usually moderately uncomfortable.	Very important to assess cancers of throat, larynx, mouth or nasal passages, and monitor effects of treatment.
Gastroscopy/ Endoscopy	Flexible tube is passed down esophagus (gullet) into stomach and top part of the duodenum.	Usually under heavy sedation or general anesthetic.	Important test in assessing abnormalities in the esophagus and stomach.
Cystoscopy	Very thin flexible tube is passed through urethra into the bladder.	Usually under heavy sedation or general anesthetic.	Routine test for assessing tumors of the bladder (and for treating many of them).

Test	How It Works	What It's Like	How It Helps
3. Tests Used to Look Directly at a Tumor or Organ			
Laparoscopy	Thin tube is passed through a small incision (usually near the umbilicus) into the abdominal cavity to view abdomen and pelvis. Biopsies are often taken.	Usually under general anesthetic.	Important test in assessing many cancers including ovary.
Mediastinoscopy	Thin tube is passed through a small incision low down in the neck to view lymph glands and other structures in the middle of the chest (between the lungs).	Usually under general anesthetic.	Often important in staging lung cancer and some other tumors.
4. Other Routine Tests			
ECG	Routine recording of the electrical activity of the heart.	Painless. A set of little pads are taped to your chest, wrists, and ankles.	Often done as baseline assessment before treatment starts (particularly if treatment might affect the heart).

Test	How It Works	What It's Like	How It Helps
4. Other Routine Tests			
EEG	Routine recording of the electrical activity of the brain.	Painless. A set of little pads are taped to various positions around your scalp.	Sometimes used if there are episodes of loss of consciousness that might be seizures.
MUGA	A scan measures the percentage of blood in the heart that is ejected with each heart-beat = (roughly) the strength of the heartbeat.	You get a small injection and then lie under a cam-era that scans you.	A few chemother-apy drugs (and some other things) can weaken the strength of the heartbeat. This test can detect that early. Often a "baseline" MUGA is done to see how strong your heartbeat is before treatment starts.

Table 4. Some Examples of Cancers in which Surgical Staging Is Often Recommended

Part of the Body	Operation involves	Why it is important
Breast	Axillary node sampling (or dissection or sentinel node biopsy): removing some of the lymph nodes from the armpit to see if the cancer has spread to them.	Treatment plans are different if the nodes in the armpit do have cancer in them: chemotherapy is more likely to be recommended.
Bowel	Removal and accurate assessment of the primary tumor, sampling the lymph nodes in various areas near the bowel, and often other areas as well.	Treatment plans are different if the nodes are involved—in many situations, chemotherapy has been shown to be of benefit.
Lung	(In some types of lung cancer) removal of the primary tumor and sampling if the lymph nodes in the middle of the chest (mediastinum).	Treatment (including chemotherapy and/or radiation therapy) is different depending on the extent of the primary and any involvement of nodes.
Ovary	Removal of both ovaries, Fallopian tubes, and uterus, sampling of several other areas including the lining of the abdomen (peritoneum) and samples of fluid from the abdomen (ascites).	Accurate staging cannot be done without this operation, and treatment plans depend on accurate assessment of tumor spread.
Testicle	In some cases, surgical sampling of the lymph nodes in the pelvis is important. In many cases it is not needed because the treatment plan won't be affected by it.	Treatment plans may sometimes depend on the exact assessment of nodes—in many cases this may not be needed and blood tests for tumor markers are all that is required.

Table 5. Some Examples of the Seven Basic Treatment Strategies

1. Biopsy only required	2. Tumor still present: more surgery required	3. Tumor still present: radiotherapy and/or chemotherapy required	4. No tumor present but adjuvant radio-therapy helpful
Bladder	Cervix (some)	Anus	Breast
Cervix (early)	Esophagus	Bladder	Brain
Common skin	Endometrium	Brain	Colon (some)
Lip (some)	Head & neck (most)	Choriocarcinoma	Endometrium (some)
Melanoma (some)	Liver	Colon, rectum	Esophagus
Penis	Lung (non-small-cell)	Endometrium, ovary	Head & neck (most)
Thyroid	Non-seminoma	Esophagus	Lung
Vulva (some)	Ovary	Head & neck (some)	Ovary (some)
Thyroid	Penis	Leukemia	Pancreas (some)
Vulva (some)	Sarcoma	Lung	Prostate (some)
	Stomach	Lymphoma	Rectum
	Vagina	Myeloma	Sarcoma
	Vulva	Pancreas, bile ducts	Stomach
		Prostate, penis,	Vulva, vagina, penis (some)
		Sarcoma soft tissue and bone	
		Stomach	
		Thyroid (some)	
		Urethra, ureter, kidney	

5. No tumor present but adjuvant drug therapy (chemo/hormones/biologics) helpful	6. Watchful waiting	7. Treatment for symptom control
Bladder (some)	Brain tumors (some)	(A) Symptoms from irremovable local tumor
Breast (most)	Chronic lymphocytic leukemia	Most cancer sites
Colon (most)	Eye tumors (some)	(B) Symptoms from sites of distant spread
Esophagus, pancreas	Prostate	All cancer sites
Head & neck (some)		
Kidney		
Lung (non-small-cell)		
Melanoma		
Ovary (most)		
Prostate (some)		
Rectum (most)		
Sarcomas		
Stomach (some)		
Testicular		
Urether, urethra		

Table 6. Common Drugs and Routes of Administration

Drugs Given by Mouth	Drugs Given by Injection	Drugs That Can Be Given by Mouth or Injection
Capecitabine	Alemtuzumab	Busulfan
Chlorambucil	Asparaginase	Cyclophosphamide
Erlotinib	Bevacizumab	Etoposide (VP-16)
Gefitinib	Bleomycin	Fludarabine
Hydroxyurea	Bortezomib	Melphalan
Imatinib	Carmustine	Methotrexate
Procarbazine	Cetuximab	
Temozolamide	Cisplatin, carboplatin	
Thalidomide	Cladribine	
Tretinoin	Cytarabine	
	Dacarbazine	
	Doxorubicin, epirubicin	
	Fluorouracil	
	Gemcitabine	
	Ifosfamide	
	Interferon Alfa	
	Interleukin-2	
	Irinotecan	
	Mitomycin	
	Mitoxantrone	
	Oxaliplatin	
	Paclitaxel, docetaxel	
	Pemetrexed	
	Pentostatin	
	Rituximab	
	Topotecan	
	Trastuzumab	
	Vincristine, vinblastine	
	Vinorelbine	

Hormone Therapy	Others
Tamoxifen	Goserelin acetate (Zoladex), leuprolide (Lupron): monthly injections under the skin of the abdomen
Aromatase inhibitors (letrozole, anastrozole, etc.)	BCG, mitomycin: injections into the bladder for local treatment
Flutamide Bicalutamide Megestrol	

Table 7. How Much Nausea Is Caused by the Most Commonly Used Chemotherapy Drugs

Cause little or no nausea	Cause moderate to severe nausea and/or vomiting Moderate → → → → Severe	
Anastrozole	Alemtuzumab	Carboplatin ($\geq$1 g/m^2)*
Bicalutamide	Altretamine	Carmustine ($\geq$200 mg/m^2)*
Bleomycin		Cisplatin ($\geq$70 mg/m^2)*
Busulfan	Asparaginase	Cyclophosphamide IV (>1000 mg/m^2)*
Capecitabine	Bevacizumab	Cytarabine (>1000 mg/m^2)*
Cetuximab	Carboplatin (<1000 mg/m^2)*	Dacarbazine ($\geq$500 mg/m^2)*
Chlorambucil (PO)	Carmustine (<200 mg/m^2)*	Dactinomycin
Cladribine	Cisplatin (<70 mg/m^2)*	Doxorubicin ($\geq$60 mg/m^2)*

Cause little or no nausea	Cause moderate to severe nausea and/or vomiting Moderate → → → → Severe	
Cyclophosphamide (PO)	Cyclophosphamide IV ($\leq$1000 mg/m^2)*	Doxorubicin IV bolus
Cytarabine (<200 mg/m^2)*	Cytarabine (200–1000 mg/m^2)*	Epirubicin ($\geq$90 mg/m^2)*
Docetaxel	Dacarbazine (<500 mg/m^2)*	Interleukin-2 (Infusion)
Erlotinib	Daunorubicin	Lomustine ($\geq$60 mg/m^2)*
Estramustine	Doxorubicin (<60 mg/m^2)*	Mechlorethamine
Etoposide (<150 mg/m^2 IV and all PO)*	Epirubicin (<90 mg/m^2)*	Methotrexate (>1000 mg/m^2)*
Fludarabine	Etoposide ($\geq$150 mg/m^2)*	Pemetrexed
Fluorouracil	Idarubicin	Streptozocin
Flutamide	Imatinib	Thiotepa (high doses used for allogeneic stem cell transplants)
Gefitinib	Ifosfamide	Gemcitabine
Hydroxyurea	Melphalan	Interferon
Irinotecan (CPT-11)	Goserelin	Lomustine (<60 mg/m^2)*
Letrozole	Mitoxantrone	Leuprolide
Mercaptopurine	Temozolomide	
Methotrexate (250–1000 mg/m^2)*	Interleukin-2 (SQ)	Mitomycin
Methotrexate (<250 mg/m^2)*	Topotecan	
Pentostatin	Levamisole	Procarbazine

Cause little or no nausea	Cause moderate to severe nausea and/or vomiting Moderate → → → → Severe	
Oxaliplatin		
Paclitaxel		
Rituximab		
Teniposide		
Thioguanine		
Tretinoin		
Trastuzumab (Herceptin*)		
Vinblastine		
Vincristine		
Vinorelbine		

* The symbol "/m²" means the dose is adjusted to your body surface area (per square meter). The average is around 1.75 m² so these doses will be multiplied accordingly.

Table 8. Antinauseants

Name of Drug or Type of Drug	Example of Brand Name	Usually Given by....	Notes
Metoclopramide	Reglan	TABLET OR INJECTION	Inhibits the CTZ & empties the stomach.
Prochlorperazine	Compazine	TABLET, SUPPOSITORY OR INJECTION	Acts on a part of the brain to reduce nausea.
H3 Blockers (e.g., ondansetron, granisetron)	Zofran Kytril	TABLETS OR INJECTION	Very powerful for use with chemotherapy that causes a lot of nausea, or if other antinausea medications not working. Only effective in first two or three days—no use later.
Steroids (e.g., dexamethasone)	Decadron	TABLETS OR INJECTION	Mechanism unknown—works best in patients with delayed nausea (many days after chemotherapy).
Scopolamine	Transderm-Scōp	SKIN PATCHES	Acts on part of brain to reduce nausea.

Name of Drug or Type of Drug	Example of Brand Name	Usually Given by....	Notes
"Over the counter" antinauseants	Gravol	TABLETS OR SUPPOSITORIES	Are not meant to work when others don't—but occasionally can be wonderfully helpful!
"Anti-side-effects" treatment	Benadryl	TABLET OR INJECTION	Not an antinauseant—but may be given to reduce the chance of reactions to some chemotherapy (eg., paclitaxel) such as: skin rashes, severely lowered blood pressure or slow heartbeat.
Lorazepam	Ativan	TABLETS	Can be used night before to calm down patients anxious about chemotherapy. Also a sedative. Also decreases memory of nausea.

Table 9. Hair Loss with Some of the More Commonly Used Chemotherapy Drugs

Drugs Which Almost Always Cause Hair Loss	Drugs Which May Cause Hair Loss	Drugs Which Rarely Cause Hair Loss
Adriamycin (doxorubicin)	Cyclophosphamide	Platinum
Epirubicin	5-Fluorouracil	Vincristine
VP-16	Vinblastine	Bleomycin
Mechlorethamine		Methotrexate
Procarbazine		Mitomycin
Actinomycin-D		Mitoxantrone
Taxol		Melphalan

Table 10. Other Effects of Some Chemotherapy Drugs

Sense of Taste	Food tastes peculiar or metallic	Large number of drugs can do this
Hearing	Loss of high-tone hearing, buzzing in ears	Platinum drugs (cisplatin, carboplatin)
Nerves	Numbness or tingling in toes and fingers (occasionally with weakness)	Vincristine, bortezomib, cisplatin, docetaxel, oxaliplatin, paclitaxel
Motility of Bowel	Bloated abdomen and no bowel action	Vincristine, busulfan, pemetrexed, temozolamide, thalidomide, vinorelbine
Kidney	Usually effects do not cause symptoms but blood tests show toxicity	Cisplatin, carboplatin

Skin Pigment	Darkening of skin folds, sometimes mouth	Bleomycin, doxorubicin, hydroxyurea, cyclophosphamide, procarbazine
Strength of Heartbeat	Breathlessness, particularly made worse when lying down	Doxorubicin, daunorubicin, epirubicin, mitoxantrone, trastuzumab
Fertility	Inability to start a pregnancy	Many drugs (and many tumors) may stop fertility—ask your doctor
Fetus	Abnormalities of fetus as it grows	Again, many drugs are potentially capable of this—so if you intend to start a pregnancy (or have started one) make sure your doctor knows.
White Blood Cells	Signs of infection/fever, chills, cough	Most chemotherapy drugs
Hair	Hair loss	See Table 9 on Hair Loss
Mouth	Mouth sores	Most chemotherapy drugs
Hand/Foot	Redness, tenderness, numbness, tingling, and peeling of palms and soles	Capecitabine, liposomal daunorubicin, fluorouracil, oxaliplatin, docetaxel

Table 11. A Few of the Current Generation of Biologics

Formal or "chemical" name	Proprietary (brand) name	Target molecule that the biologic is aimed at	Situations in which the biologic can be used	Most common side effects
bevacizumab	Avastin	A-VEGF	Colo-rectal, (under trial in others)	More common: high blood pressure, nausea and vomiting, headache, tiredness, diarrhea, mouth sores, loss of appetite
alemtuzumab	Campath	CD 52	B-CLL, transplant	More common: increased risk of infection (fever, chills, cough), tiredness, lightheadedness, nausea and vomiting
cetuximab	Erbitux	EGFR	Colo-rectal, liver	More common: rash, tiredness, diarrhea, mouth sores, cough and trouble breathing

Formal or "chemical" name	Proprietary (brand) name	Target mole-cule that the biologic is aimed at	Situations in which the bio-logic can be used	Most common side effects
imatinib	Gleevec	Selective TK inhibitor	GIST, CML, glioma	More common: nausea and vomiting, diarrhea, indigestion, headache, muscle cramps, skin rash
trastuzumab	Herceptin	EGF-R	Her2 positive breast	More common: increased risk of infection (fever, chills, cough), diar-rhea, nausea, and vomiting
gefitinib	Iressa	EGF-R	Lung (some)	More common: diarrhea, rash, dry skin, itchy skin, nausea. Less common: dry mouth, fatigue, vom-iting, eye problems
pertuzumab	Omnitarg	HER2	Undergoing clinical trails	Data unavailable at present

Formal or "chemical" name	Proprietary (brand) name	Target molecule that the biologic is aimed at	Situations in which the biologic can be used	Most common side effects
rituximab	Rituxan	CD 20	lymphoma	More common: increased risk of infection (fever, chills, cough), nausea and vomiting, fatigue, light-headedness
erlotinib	Tarceva	EGF-TK	Lung (some), pancreas	More common: diarrhea, rash, dry skin, itchy skin, nausea and vomiting. Less common: dry and sore mouth, fatigue, eye problems (blurred vision, redness or pain), loss of appetite

Formal or "chemical" name	Proprietary (brand) name	Target molecule that the biologic is aimed at	Situations in which the biologic can be used	Most common side effects
bortezomib	Velcade	Proteasome inhibitor	Myeloma	More common: fatigue, increased risk of infection (fever, chills, cough), nausea, diarrhea, constipation, rash, insomnia/ sleepiness, numbness/ tingling in fingers and toes
ibritumomab	Zevalin	CD 20	Some lymphomas	More common: increased risk of infection (fever, chills, cough), tiredness, nausea, lowered blood pressure

"Where Can I Get More Help?"

A Directory of Organizations, Sources & Websites

General Cancer Websites:

American Cancer Society
http://www.cancer.org/

The website for this US community-based voluntary health organization provides current awareness for new cancer treatment developments and detailed information on a wide variety of different cancers.

American Institute for Cancer Research Online
http://www.aicr.org/

The American Institute for Cancer Research is a leading national charity in the field of diet, nutrition and cancer prevention. The information you'll find here could help you begin to reduce cancer risk for you and your family.

Coalition of National Cancer Cooperative Groups
http://www.cancertrialshelp.org

This network of cancer clinical trials specialists includes cooperative groups, cancer centers, academic medical centers, community hospitals, physician practices and patient advocate groups, representing the interests of more than 17,000 cancer investigators, hundreds of patient advocates, and thousands of patients worldwide. It offers programs and information for physicians, patient advocate groups, and patients that are designed to increase awareness of and participation in cancer clinical trials.

MayoClinic.com
http://www.mayoclinic.com/health/cancer/CA99999

The Mayo Clinic's website offers information on cancer in general and more detailed topics such as types of cancer, symptoms, resources, treatments and research. It also offers a drug database with extensive and useful information for patients.

National Cancer Institute
http://www.cancer.gov/

This service, from the National Institutes of Health (NIH), acts as a gateway for the most recent and accurate information on cancer. This site provides information on types of cancer, treatment, clinical trials, genetics, causes, risk factors, prevention, testing, coping, etc.

Oncolink

http://www.oncolink.com/

Founded in 1994 by the University of Pennsylvania, this sites provides comprehensive information about specific types of cancer, updates on cancer treatments, news about research advances, and more.

University of Texas M.D. Anderson Cancer Center

http://www.manderson.org

The M.D. Anderson Cancer Center is located at the University of Texas in Houston. It is devoted exclusively to cancer patient care, research, education and prevention. M.D. Anderson is one of three comprehensive cancer centers designated by the National Act of 1971 and one of 39 comprehensive cancer centers today. Their website provides extensive information on different types of cancer and cancer prevention, patient stories, online audio and video presentations, and links to other useful sites.

General Cancer Books:

Buchholz, Susie and William Buchholz. *Live Longer, Live Larger: A Holistic Approach for Cancer Patients and Their Families*. Sebastopol: O'Reilly & Associates, 2001.

Cukier, Daniel and Virginia E. McCullough. *Coping with Radiation Therapy*. Los Angeles: Lowell House, 2001.

Dorfman, Elena and Heidi Schultz Adams. *Here and Now: Inspirational Stories of Cancer Survivors*. New York: Marlowe & Company, 2001.

Harpham, Wendy Schlessel. *Diagnosis: Cancer: Your Guide to the First Months of Healthy Survivorship*. New York: W.W. Norton & Company, 2003.

Hunter, Brenda. *Staying Alive: Life-Changing Strategies for Surviving Cancer*. Colorado Springs: WaterBrook Press, 2004.

Jevne, Ronna. *Hoping, Coping & Moping: Handling Life When Illness Makes It Tough*. Los Angeles: Health Information Press, 2000.

Kelvin, Joanne F. and Leslie B. Tyson. *100 Questions & Answers about Cancer Symptoms and Cancer Treatment Side Effects*. Sudbury, MA: Jones and Bartlett Publishers, 2005.

McGinn, Kerry Anne and Pamela J. Haylock. *Women's Cancers: How to Prevent Them, How to Treat Them, How to Beat Them*. Alameda, CA: Hunter House, 2003.

Thomas, Lucy, Nancy Oster, and Darol Joseff. *Making Informed Medical Decisions*. Sebastopol: O'Reilly & Associates, 2000.

Acknowledgements

The idea for this book was Dr. Pam Catton's.

Pam is a radiation oncologist at the Princess Margaret Hospital and the head of its Patient Education unit. The prospect of working with her on projects like this one was the main reason for my wanting to move there a few years ago.

Pam wanted us to write a real and practical navigational aid for the cancer patient and family, and has been involved at every stage of this book from the first notes to the final manuscript. I cannot overstate how important her contribution has been to this book from the very beginning.

Anna Porter, founder of Key Porter Books, got the idea of this book immediately, and it was she who thought that the original subtitle of the book would make a much better title. (Since we have followed her advice, we hope she is right.)

It was Linda Pruessen at Key Porter who suggested that we limit ourselves to writing a guide to get the reader through the first few weeks.

Clare McKeon—with whom I have worked on several of my books for Key Porter—is the best editor a writer could wish for. She is simply wonderful: creative, flexible, patient, and generous (particularly when an author is behind on his deadlines).

At the Princess Margaret Hospital pharmacy I had a lot of assistance from Pamela Ng and Caroline Como.

My wife, Dr. Patricia Shaw, is an internationally known pathologist (also at the Princess Margaret Hospital) specializing and doing research in ovarian cancer. Pat helped me through a lot of the details of pathology and of molecular markers. It is mainly due to her clear thinking about the relationship between the way a cancer can be identified (by its appearance and its molecular markers) and the way it is likely to behave, that I found that I am not as bad at pathology as I feared (though not yet as good as I hoped).